Ketogenic Cookbook

500 Easy Low-Carb Weight Loss Recipes

Abel Jones

Table of Contents

Introduction 17

Chapter 1 19

How to Get Started: Transitioning Into Ketosis 19

The "Standard American Diet" vs. Keto Diet 19

Entering Ketosis 20

Chapter 2 21

Fats and Oils 21

Protein 21

Dairy 21

Vegetables 22

Fruits 22

Drinks 22

Others 22

Food List by Color 23

Green List 23

Orange List 25

Red List 26

Ketogenic Diet Foods and their Macros 27

Chapter 3 31

Creating Your Own Meal Plan 31

Helpful Tips for the Ketogenic Diet 31

4 Week Keto Meal Plan 33

Chapter 4: Breakfasts 37

Keto Pancakes and Syrup 38

Bacon Avocado Breakfast Muffins 39

Orange Cinnamon Scones 40

Red Pepper, Mozzarella and Bacon Frittata 41

Cheese and Sausage Pies 42

Breakfast Quiche 43

Chicharrones con Huevos (Pork Rind and Eggs) 44

Raspberry & Cacao Breakfast Bowl 45

Anaheim Pepper Gruyere Waffles 46

Nutty Cocoa Cereal 47

Breakfast Tacos 48

Cheesy Bacon and Chive Omelet 49

Pizza Waffles 50

Anchovy, Spinach and Asparagus Omelet 51

Autumn Keto Pumpkin Bread 52

Keto Oatmeal 53

Batter Coated Cheddar Cheese 54

Mahón Kale Sausage Omelet Pie 55

Monterey Bacon-Scallions Omelet 56

— Smoked Turkey Bacon and Avocado Muffins 57

Hot n' Spicy Scramble 58

Chorizo Breakfast Peppers 59

Breakfast Bread Pudding 60

Creamy Chocó & Avocado Mousse 61

Sour Cream Cheese Pancakes 62

Vesuvius Scrambled Eggs with Provolone 63

— Adorable Pumpkin Flaxseed Muffins 64

Baked Ham and Kale Scrambled Eggs 65

Bell Pepper and Ham Omelet 66

Chia Flour Pancakes 67

Chocó Mocha Chia Porridge 68

Crimini Mushroom with Boiled Eggs Breakfast 69

Egg Whites and Spinach Omelet 70

Fast Protein and Peanut-Butter Pancakes 71

Hemp Muffins with Walnuts 72

Keto Baked Pancetta and Eggs 73

Keto Bilberry Coconut Mush.. 74

Keto French Almond Toast 75

Pork and Sage Breakfast Burgers.. 76

Quick Coconut Berry Pancakes... 77

Tomato Basil & Chili Scramble.. 78

Mediterranean Egg Scramble 79

Millet Gingerbread Mash.. 80

Scrambled Eggs with Bacon and Gouda Cheese.................................... 81

Nutty Cinnamon Granola.. 82

Baked Buckwheat Pancakes with Hazelnuts 83

Baked Parmesan-Almond Zucchini.. 84

Eggs with Motley Peppers and Zucchini... 85

Kale, Peppers and Crumbled Feta Omelet 86

Mini Ham Omelettes Muffins 87

Nonpareil Bacon Waffles.. 88

Power Greens and Sausage Casserole... 89

Simple Bacon Pepper Pot 90

Spinach-Chard Puree with Almonds 91

Buttermilk Seed Rusk's 92

Ketogenic Mug Bread 93

Lemon Cheesecake Breakfast Mousse 94

Cacao and Raspberry Pudding... 95

Mozzarella, Red Pepper & Bacon Frittata 96

Rosemary, Sausage & Cheese Pies 97

Pump-Cakes.. 98

Protein Loaded French bread 99

Fisherman's Breakfast 100

Herbed Eggs.. 101

Smoked Salmon and Avocado Breakfast 102

Creamy Greens Breakfast Pie 103

Sausage Biscuits.. 104

Olives and Avocado Frittata 105

Cheesy Cauliflower Waffle 106

Eggs n' Steak Breakfast 107

Keto Breakfast Biscuit 108

Bacon Hash and Eggs 109

Bacon Waffles 110

Ham and Cheese Omelet 111

Egg-Stuffed Meat Balls 112

Cheeseburger Quiche 113

Vegan-Friendly Scramble 114

Bacon and Peanut Butter Muffin Cups 115

Sweet, Salty, and Savory Crepe 116

Eggs Benedict 117

Almond Bread 118

Chapter 5: Poultry **119**

Chicken Pie 120

Classic Chicken Parmigiana 121

Turkey Leg Roast 122

Slow-Cooked Greek Chicken 123

Roasted Bacon-Wrapped Chicken 124

Crispy Curried Chicken 125

The Perfect Baked Chicken Wings 126

Chicken in Kung Pao Sauce 127

Chicken BBQ Pizza 128

Slow Cooked Chicken Masala 129

Baked Buttered Chicken 130

Chicken, Bacon & Cream Cheese Pot Pie 131

Chicken Hash 132

Chicken Parmesan 133

Chicken Stir-Fry 134

Nacho Chicken Casserole 135

Kung Pao Chicken 136

Chipotle Blackberry Wings 137

Jalapeno Chicken Casserole 138

Roasted Turkey Legs 139

Asian Grilled Chicken 140

Fettuccine Chicken Alfredo 141

Ethiopian Doro Watt 142

Buffalo Chicken 143

Curried Coconut Chicken Fingers 144

Greek Chicken 145

Chicken Satay 146

Sage and Orange Glazed Duck 147

Pad Thai 148

Creamy Tarragon Chicken 149

Chicken & Endive Casserole 150

Creamy Smoked Turkey Salad with Almonds 151

Creamy Chicken Salad 152

Duck Breast with Balsamic Vinegar 153

Zesty Herbed Chicken 154

Chicken Pesto Salad 155

Hot Peri-Peri Chicken on Green Salad 156

Mediterranean Chicken 157

Turkey Meatballs 158

Roast Chicken and Pepper Salad 159

Chicken and Cucumber Salad 160

Baked Chicken and Avocado 161

Crunchy Chicken Waldorf salad 162

Spicy Chicken Thighs 163

Blackberry and Grilled Chicken Salad 164

Chili and Lime Meatballs 165

Sour Avocado and Chicken Moussaka 166

Chicken, Bacon and Avocado Sandwich 167

Roasted Lemony Chicken & Prosciutto with Brussels sprouts 168

Pordenone Cauliflower Lasagna 169

Easy Chicken Cordon Bleu 170

"Chicken Alfredo" Pizza 171

Chicken Angel Eggs 172

Oriental Garlicky Chicken Thighs 173

Chicken and Broccoli filled Zucchini 174

Baked Creamy Cauliflower-Broccoli Chicken 175

Baked Manchego Chicken Wings 176

Bacon Chicken Patties 177

Curry-Spiced Salad 178

Chicken Paprikash 179

Chapter 6: Seafood **180**

Sweet and Sour Snapper 181

Creamy Haddock 182

Pan Fried Hake 183

Pesto and Almond Salmon 184

Lime Avocado Salmon 185

Glazed Sesame Ginger Salmon 186

Buttery Shrimp 187

Keto Friendly Sushi 188

Stuffed Avocado with Tuna 189

Herb Baked Salmon Fillets 190

Salmon with a Walnut Crust 191

Baked Glazed Salmon 192

Salmon Burgers 193

Keto Crab Sushi 194

Coco Shrimps and Chili Dip 195

Tuna/Smoked Salmon Salad 196

Salmon Salad in Avocado Cups 197

Mackerel Salad 198

Crab Cakes 199

Shrimp & Avocado Salad 200

Salmon Salad in Avo Cups 201

Tuna Avocado Bites 202

Thai Fish Curry 203

Chapter 7: Meat **204**

Hearty Portobello Burgers 205
Pork and Shrimp Stuffed Peppers 206
Spiced Beef 207
Sirloin Tip Cut with Cilantro Sauce 208
Bacon Layered Lasagna 209
Macadamia Crusted Lamb Chops 210
Slow-Cooker Stroganoff 211
Spicy Mexican Meatballs 212
Bell Peppers Stuffed 213
Keto Burger Patties 214
Meatballs in Coconut Broth 215
Sunday's Best Roast Beef 216
Apple Rosemary Pork Chops 217
Lemon Mustard Pork Loin 218
Cheesy Cauliflower and Bacon Casserole 219
Seared Ribeye Steak 220
Poblano Peppers Stuffed with Pork 221
Crispy Slow Roasted Pork Shoulder 222
Italian Style Meatballs 223
Grilled Asian Short Ribs 224
Cheeseburger Waffles 225
Slow Cooker Beef with Dried Herbs 226
Lamb Cutlets with Garlic Sauce 227
Hot Mexican Meatballs 228
Baked Cheesy Meatballs 229
Tangy Asian Short Ribs 230
Beanless Chili con Carne 231
Delicious Meaty Meatloaf 232
Pulled Pork Shoulder 233
Slow Roast Lamb 234
Lamb Curry & Spinach 235
Cheeseburger Casserole 236
Leftover Meat Salad 237

Asian-Flavored Steak 238

Stir Fried Beef 239

Pizza on Lettuce Rolls 240

Spicy Bacon-Wrapped Dogs 241

Spring Roll in a Bowl 242

Homemade Meatballs 243

Beef Shred Salad 244

Cheesy Hotdog Pockets 245

Cheese Steak Salad 246

Sausage and Cheese Balls 247

Bunless Bacon and Almond Butter Burger 248

Pigs in a Blanket 249

Cheesy Crust Pizza 250

No-Bread Cheeseburger 251

Ham and Cheese Stromboli 252

Squash Spaghetti Lasagna Dish 253

Spicy Italian Sausage and Spinach Casserole 254

Mediterranean Pecorino Romano Breaded Cutlets 255

Pumpkin Chili 256

Monterey Jack Steak 257

Cheesy Keto Pizza 258

Sausage & Cheese Bombs 259

Spicy Spinach Casserole 260

Bolognese Squash Spaghetti 261

Baked Pork Chops in Sweet-Sour Marinade 262

Grilled Cheese and Ham Sandwich 263

Beef Sausage, Bacon & Broccoli Casserole 264

Cheesy Bacon Spinach Log 265

Savoury Mince 266

Chorizo Stuffed Bell Peppers 267

Sour Sausages with Shallots and Kalamata Olives 268

Sour and Spicy Goat Skewers 269

Meaty Bagels 270

Madras Lamb Curry 271

Balsamic Pork.. 272

Bolognese Mince 273

Smoky Pork Cassoulet.. 274

Tomato Bredie 275

Chapter 8 Soups & Stews.. **276**

Lemon Chicken Stew 277

Beef Chuck Cabbage Stew 278

Hearty Beef Stew 279

Curried Chicken Stew... 280

Curried Cauliflower & Chicken Stew.. 281

Farmhouse Lamb & Cabbage Stew.. 282

Seafood Stew 283

Rosemary Garlic Beef Stew... 284

Creamy Chicken & Pumpkin Stew 285

The Best Beef Stew 286

Thai Nut Chicken... 287

Bouillabaisse Fish Stew 288

Spanish Chorizo Soup 289

Beef & Broccoli Stew 290

Mussel Stew... 291

Sweet Potato Stew 292

Oxtail Stew.. 293

Italian Gnocchi Soup... 294

Loaded Cauliflower Soup.. 295

French Onion Soup 296

Thai Chicken Soup... 297

Curried Cauliflower Soup.. 298

Easy Everyday Chicken Soup... 299

Creamy Chicken & Tomato Soup... 300

Tomato & Basil Soup 301

Beef & Cabbage Soup 302

3 Ingredients Vegetable Beef Soup 303

Clam Chowder 304

Mushroom Soup 305

Seafood Soup 306

Cream of Broccoli & Mushroom Soup 307

Beef & Vegetable Soup 308

Cream of Carrot Soup 309

Cream of Tomato Soup 310

Creamy Zucchini Soup 311

Indian Curried Cauliflower Soup 312

Broccoli & Blue cheese Soup 313

Italian Meatball Zoodle Soup 314

BBQ Chicken Soup 315

Super-Fast Egg Drop Soup 316

Spicy Slow-Cooked Chicken Soup 317

BBQ Pizza Soup 318

Cheese and Bacon Soup 319

Beef Cabbage Parsley Soup 320

Boneless Lamb Stew 321

Keto Butternut Squash Soup 322

Spinach Soup with Almonds and Parmesan 323

Keto Light Cabbage Soup 324

Oriental Shrimp Soup 325

Zucchini Soup with Crunchy Cured Ham 326

Hot Chili Soup 327

Jalapeno Popper Soup 328

Cheeseburger Soup 329

Malaysian Bone Broth Soup 330

Cheeseburger Soup Indulgence 331

Cabbage with Ground Beef Stew 332

Slow Cooker Roast and Chicken Stew 333

Italian Fish Stew 334

Chicken and Mushroom Stew 335

Beef Shin Stew 336

Tuna Fish Stew 337
Cauliflower and Cheese Chowder 338
Chicken Bacon Chowder 339
Chapter 9: Vegetable Recipes 340
Squash Carbonara 341
Ratatouille 342
Cauliflower Bake 343
Caulicake 344
Spiced Kale "Meatballs" 345
Pumpkin Carbonara 346
One Pot Italian Sausage Meal 347
No-Sweat Spinach Salad 348
Baked Cheesy Zucchini 349
Level-Up Spinach Salad 350
Pizza in Mushroom Cups 351
Hearty Salad 352
Spinach and Goat Cheese Salad 353
Greek Eggplant Salad 354
Egg and Avocado Salad 355
Tricolor Salad 356
Cucumber Strawberry Salsa and Grilled Halloumi 357
Green Veggie Salad 358
Bacon, Lettuce, Tomato Salad 359
Broccoli Salad 360
Bacon with Cheesy Cauliflower Mash 361
Creamed Spinach 362
Cheesy Zoodles with Fresh Basil 363
Veggie Burger Patties 364
Mascarpone Zucchini Rolls 365
Tasty Cauliflower Rice 366
Roquefort Spinach, Zoodles and Bacon Salad 367
Spinach and Cheese Stuffed Mushrooms 368
Baked Broccoli with Mushrooms and Parmesan 369

Ail Creamy Brussels sprouts 370

Spicy Cauliflower with Sujuk Sausages 371

Chapter 10: Desserts & Fat Bombs **372**

All-stars Peanut-Butter Cookies 373

Almond Chocolate Brownies 374

Almond Chocolate Cookies... 375

Carrot Muffins 376

Coconut Jelly Cake 377

Cottage Pumpkin Pie Ice Cream 378

Divine Keto Chocolate Biscotti 379

Halloween Pumpkin Ice Cream 380

Homemade Nut Bars 381

Chia Seed Cream... 382

Hemp and Chia Seeds Cream 382

Chocolate Brownies... 383

Chocolate Pecan Bites 384

Creamy Chocolate Mousse.. 384

Hazelnut Chocolate Cream 385

Lemon Coconut Pearls... 385

Instant Coffee Ice Cream 386

Jam "Eye" Cookies 387

Lime & Vanilla Cheesecake... 388

Strawberry Pudding... 389

Kiwi Fiend Ice Cream 390

Minty Avocado Lime Sorbet 391

Morning Zephyr Cake 392

Peanut Butter Balls.. 393

Pecan Flax Seed Blondies 394

Peppermint Chocolate Ice Cream... 395

Puff-up Coconut Waffles 396

Raspberry Chocolate Cream 397

Raw Cacao Hazelnut Cookies.. 398

Sinless Pumpkin Cheesecake Muffins 399

Sour Hazelnuts Biscuits with Arrowroot Tea 400
Tartar Keto Cookies 401
Wild Strawberries Ice Cream 402
Mini Lemon Cheesecakes 402
Chocolate Layered Coconut Cups 403
Pumpkin Pie Chocolate Cups 404
Fudgy Cake 405
Easy Sticky Chocolate Fudge 406
Raspberry & Coconut Fat Bombs 407
Strawberry Cheesecake Ice Cream Cups 408
Buttery Pecan Delights 408
Peppermint Patties 409
Chocolate Fudge 410
Cinna-Bun Balls 411
Vanilla Mousse Cups 412
Rich & Creamy Fat Bomb Ice Cream 413
English Toffee Treats 414
Fudgy Peanut Butter Squares 415
Lemon Squares & Coconut Cream 416
Rich Almond Butter Cake & Chocolate Sauce 417
Peanut Butter Cake Covered in Chocolate Sauce 418

Chapter 11: Savory Snacks **419**

Greek-Style Fat Bomb Balls 420
Bacon & Onion Cookie Bites 421
Guacamole & Bacon Fat Bombs 422
Bacon and Egg Fat Bombs 423
Simple Parmesan Crisps 424
Mini Pizza Bombs 425
Cheesy Bacon Fat Bombs 425
Smoked Turkey, Blue Cheese Eggs 426
Double Cheese Artichoke Dip 427
Easy Artichokes 427
Pancetta & Eggs 428

— Parmesan, Herb & Sun-dried Tomato Bombs 429

Cauliflower Tater Tots 430

Keto Margherita Pizza 431

Easy Peasy Cheese Pizza 432

Keto Trio Queso Quesadilla 433

Bacon and Cheese Melt 434

BLT Roll 434

Portobello Pizza 435

Basil and Bell Pepper Pizza 436

Chapter 12: Smoothies 437

Blueberry Almond Smoothie 438

Choco-Cashew Orange Smoothie 438

Strawberry Majoram Smoothie 439

The Green Fuel 439

Beet Cucumber Smoothie 440

Green Devil Smoothie 440

Cilantro and Ginger Smoothie 441

Green Coconut Smoothie 441

Green Dream Keto Smoothie 442

Almond Choc Shake 442

Keto Celery and Nut Smoothie 443

Coco and Blueberry Smoothie 443

Lime Peppermint Smoothie 444

Berry Breakfast Shake 444

Red Grapefruit Kale Smoothies 445

Simple Keto Avocado Smoothie 445

Vanilla Protein Smoothie 446

Keto Avocado Smoothie 446

Caramel Coffee Smoothie 447

Creamy Chocolate Milk 447

Conclusion... 448

Introduction

That burning sensation in your chest after climbing up two flights of stairs, jeans that don't fit, and friends that tell you "I think you're getting chubby,"— are you getting a bit tired of these? Are you in dire need of losing those excess pounds you've carried around since Thanksgiving three years ago?

Right now, maybe you're feeling awful about your weight and physical appearance, but let me tell you this: the moment that you decided that you need to do something about your dilemma (like downloading this book), means you're already halfway to losing weight, improving your health, and becoming a better version of you.

But before I introduce this effective and revolutionary diet that will help solve your problems, let's straighten a few things up. Let me ask you a few fundamental questions that may just shift your perspective:

What is the real reason why you want to shed the fat and lose weight? Is it to boost your confidence and have the perfect bikini body? Or is it so that you can run that marathon you have always wanted to?

You see, there's nothing wrong with wanting to lose weight in order to become more attractive, but should this be your main focus?

This may be your initial goal, but after committing to the Ketogenic lifestyle, you will soon realize that the benefits are far more extensive than just mere weight loss.

Mood stabilization, hormone regulation, slowed ageing, blood sugar balance, memory and cognitive improvement...these are just a few of the profound changes your body will embrace, should you choose to follow the advice that is contained in the pages to follow.

So, besides achieving a "desirable" body, your main purpose will rapidly shift to becoming a healthy, energetic person, avoiding the severe complications of being overweight or obese.

The World Health Organization (WHO) defines overweight and obesity as an "abnormal or excessive fat accumulation that **may** impair health." Experts have recognized that the primary cause of these conditions is a deadly combination of an unhealthy diet plus a sedentary lifestyle.

It is quite disturbing to note that over 1.9 billion adults all over the world are suffering these conditions (WHO, 2014); 42 million children below 5 years old are also either obese or overweight.

Now you might be asking: *How does this affect me?*

Well, carrying extra pounds around your mid-section puts you at great risk of developing chronic illnesses such as stroke, heart disease, type 2 diabetes, osteoarthritis, breast cancer and colon cancer, just to name a few. Although these complications may alarm you, the good news is that obesity can be reversed and the complications that go with it are preventable.

The simplest answer is invariably the correct one, and you have most likely heard it a thousand times before...

A balanced diet mixed with a healthy dose of exercise.

The first part of the statement is where most individuals slip up. The so called "balanced diet" is never fully explained and always shrouded in mystery and confusion.

Maybe you've already tried some of the fad diets that are popular right now, but they do not seem to work. Or you have also tried some of the fasting and starvation diets out there that promise instant results, but you just can't seem to keep up with the idea of skipping meals. Well, maybe it's time that you try a diet that is scientifically proven to help you burn fat, lose weight, and provide you much, much more - the Ketogenic Diet.

Also called as the Keto Diet, this food program is a low-carb high-fat diet that "forces" the body to enter into a different metabolic state where fat is burned as fuel for energy instead of glucose (I will discuss this in more detail at a later stage in the book).

You may think that the Keto Diet is a fairly new food regimen, yet another fad, but on the contrary, this diet has already become popular in the 1940's when it was used to help minimize seizures of children with epilepsy.

It has since lost its place under the spotlight when anticonvulsant drugs became more widely available to the market. It only gained popularity again in the 1990's, when the son of a famous Hollywood director used the diet to help him reduce his epileptic episodes, with remarkable results.

This paved way for further research into the Keto Diet. These studies found that a low-carb, high-fat diet was not only able to help minimize seizures for patients with epilepsy, but also help individuals to lose weight, minimize abdominal fat, increase HDL and LDL levels (good cholesterol), decrease blood sugar levels, prevent cancer and cognitive decline. So in short, this diet that I'm about to introduce to you will not only help you burn fat and lose weight, but it can also deliver other amazing benefits for your overall health!

The chapters of this book will provide you with the information on how you can start transitioning into ketosis, and how to create your own Keto meal plan. I will also provide a comprehensive list of Ketogenic approved foods. I've also included delicious Keto recipes for breakfast, lunch, dinner and snacks. Most importantly, I've included an eating plan that can help guide you on your first month in the Keto Diet.

Today is a beginning of a better and healthier you!

Chapter 1

How to Get Started: Transitioning Into Ketosis

You've heard of countless low-carb diets that help you lose weight and at the same time deliver amazing health benefits, but a low-carb high-fat diet? *How does that work? How can eating more fat help you lose fat?* Well, that is where the metabolic processes *ketosis* steps in to help out.

The "Standard American Diet" vs. Keto Diet

Ever since modern agriculture was introduced, man's normal diet has shifted from being meat and vegetable eaters (our hunter and gatherer ancestors) to individuals who eat more processed carbohydrates such as pasta, bread, rice, and potatoes.

Now, there's nothing wrong with carbs. Carbs per se aren't actually bad for our health, as long as we consume more of the healthy types of carbs such as vegetables (yes they contain carbs too), legumes, whole-grains, fruits, and nuts.

However, if you really want to lose weight and also prevent developing type 2 diabetes, then it would be advisable to limit a number of carbs you consume. That's because when you eat foods high in carbohydrates, they get broken down in your blood as glucose (sugar). This means that when you consume lots of carbs, a high amount of glucose becomes present in your blood, resulting in high blood sugar levels.

Again, carbs aren't all bad because in a normal diet, the body will reach out for glucose in order to use it as fuel for energy, as well as fuel the other functions of our body. The only problem is that any glucose that isn't used by the body as energy, will be stored as body fat. This is one of the main reasons why a lot of people in this day and age are overweight - because they consume too many carbs and only expend little of it, due to their sedentary lifestyle.

The Ketogenic Diet, on the other hand, reduces the consumption of carbs to a minimum and increases healthy fats in one's diet. When carbs are reduced, your body will naturally look for other sources to burn for energy and in this case, fats are chosen. The Ketogenic Diet shifts your body into a metabolic state called ketosis, a process that burns fat instead of glucose, allowing you to shed unwanted weight easily and quickly.

Entering Ketosis

As you now know, the target of the Ketogenic Diet is to allow your body to enter into ketosis; but the question now is, *how*?

There are three different types of Ketogenic Diets— the Standard Ketogenic Diet (SKD), Cyclical Ketogenic Diet (CKD), and the Targeted Ketogenic Diet (TKD). The latter two variants of the diet will be ignored, due to their complexity. People who have sedentary lifestyles and wish to lose weight through this diet are advised to follow the SKD. This variation recommends limiting the consumption of your carbs to 20-50 grams daily, which means your macronutrients should be made up of 70%-75% fat, 20%-25% protein, and 5%-10% carbs. The number of daily calories you can consume, however, relies on your weight, height, age, and activity. If you're unsure how to do this, you can always consult a keto calculator, which are widely available online. I recommend the one at www.ruled.me for its accuracy.

(https://www.ruled.me/keto-calculator/)

You might be a little skeptical of the Ketogenic Diet right now, especially if you think that carbs currently make up the biggest portion of your diet. Set aside your assumptions for the duration of this book and approach the next two weeks of your life like an experiment. Trust that if you consume a healthy number of calories and eat foods that are nutrient dense (ex. vegetables, and healthy fat), then you don't have to worry about "dieting" at all! You can safely enter into a state of ketosis when following the prescribed guidelines closely.

I'd like to remind you that unlike any other diets, the Keto Diet needs your complete commitment to the diet in order for you to achieve the state of ketosis. Depending on your body type, activity level, and your diet, you can get into ketosis anywhere from 2 days to a week. For beginners, it is advisable that you use urine ketone sticks (such as Ketostix) to monitor the levels of ketones in your body and ensure that you are in ketosis state. This is a useful tip to help you know whether your body is in ketosis and is burning fat as energy, apart from the other obvious indicators like an increase in energy and lack of appetite.

I must advise you, however, that before anything else, it is a must that you ask for a green light from your health care provider if you are planning to follow the Ketogenic Diet; or any type of diet for that matter. Although this diet is safe over-all, even for kids, you have to let your doctor know about this, especially if you have existing health conditions.

Pregnant women or those who are breastfeeding aren't encouraged to try the Ketogenic Diet for weight loss because this may have adverse effects on their baby.

Chapter 2

Time to purge your pantry and replace them with these Ketogenic Diet approved foods!

Fats and Oils

Since fat will make the majority of your meals, it is a must that you choose the good type (natural sources) of fat and not those that are dangerous to your health. Some of your best choices for fat are:

- Ghee or Clarified butter
- Avocado
- Coconut Oil
- Red Palm Oil
- Butter
- Coconut Butter
- Peanut Butter

- Chicken Fat
- Beef Tallow
- Non-hydrogenated Lard
- Macadamia Nuts
- Egg Yolks
- Fish rich in Omega-3 Fatty Acids like salmon, mackerel, trout, tuna, and even shellfish.

Protein

In order to achieve a state of ketosis, you need to consume 20%-25% protein in your daily caloric allowance. This means your consumption of fat will be high; carbs are low, and protein, moderate. Of course, you also want to choose the healthy sources of protein that are either organic, or grass fed.

- Meat— beef, veal, lamb, chicken, duck, pheasant, pork chops, pork loin, etc.
- Deli Meat— bacon, sausage, ham (make sure to watch out of added sugar and other fillers)
- Eggs— preferably free-range or organic eggs

- Fish— wild caught salmon, catfish, halibut, trout, tuna, etc.
- Seafood— lobster, crab, oyster, clams, mussels
- Peanut Butter—this is a great source of protein, but make sure to choose the all-natural variant

Dairy

Compared to other weight loss diets, in the Ketogenic Diet, you are encouraged to choose dairy products that are full fat. Some of the best dairy products that you can choose are:

- Hard and Soft Cheese— cream cheese, mozzarella, cheddar, etc.
- Cottage Cheese

- Heavy Whipping Cream
- Sour Cream
- Full-Fat Yogurt

Vegetables

Overall, vegetables are rich in vitamins and minerals that contribute to a healthy body. However, if you're aiming to avoid carbs, it's best that you keep away from starchy vegetables such as potatoes, yam, peas, corn, beans, and legumes. You also want to limit vegetables that taste sweet such as carrots and squash. Instead, stick with green leafy vegetables that are preferably organically grown and other low-carb veggies.

- Spinach
- Lettuce
- Collard Greens
- Mustard Greens
- Bok Choi
- Kale
- Alfalfa Sprouts
- Celery
- Tomato
- Broccoli
- Cauliflower

Fruits

Your choice of fruit is only limited to avocado and some *berries because fruits are high in carbs and sugar.

Drinks

- Water
- Black Coffee
- Herbal Tea
- Wine—white wine and dry red wine are OK, as long as they are only consumed occasionally

Others

- Homemade Mayo—if you want to buy mayo from the store, make sure that you watch out for the hidden carbs it contains
- Homemade Mustard
- Any type of Spices and Herbs
- *Honey
- *Stevia
- *Agave Nectar
- *Ketchup (Sugar-free)
- *Dark Chocolate/Cocoa

Food List by Color

Green List

This is an all-you-can-eat list - you can choose anything you like, without worrying about the carbohydrate content, as all the foods will be between 0 to 5g/100g.

It will be almost impossible to overdo your carbohydrate intake by sticking to this group of foods. Eating large amounts of protein is not recommended, so eat a moderate amount of animal protein at each meal. Include as much fat as you are comfortable with - bearing in mind that Keto is high in fat. Caution: even though these are all-you-can-eat foods, only eat when hungry, stop when full and do not overeat. The size and thickness of your palm without fingers is a good measure for a serving of animal protein. All meat, eggs, dairy, and greens should be organic, free range and grass fed where possible.

ANIMAL PROTEIN
(unless these have a rating, they are all 0g/100g)

- All eggs
- All meats, poultry, and game
- All natural and cured meats (pancetta, parma ham, capocollo etc)

- All natural and cured sausages (salami, chorizo etc)
- All offal
- All seafood (except swordfish and tilefish - high mercury content)
- Broths

DAIRY

- Cottage cheese
- Cream
- Cream cheese
- Full-cream Greek yogurt

- Full-cream milk
- Hard cheeses
- Soft cheeses

FATS

- Any rendered animal fat
- Avocado oil
- Butter
- Cheese - firm, natural, full-fat, aged cheeses (not processed)
- Coconut oil
- Duck fat
- Ghee
- Lard
- Macadamia oil

- Mayonnaise, full fat only (not from seeds oils)
- Olive oil

FLAVOURINGS AND CONDIMENTS

All flavorings and condiments are okay, provided they do not contain sugars and preservatives or vegetable (seed) oils.

NUTS AND SEEDS

- Almonds
- Flaxseeds (watch out for pre-ground flax seeds, they go rancid quickly and become toxic)
- Macadamia nuts
- Pecan nuts
- Pine nuts
- Pumpkin seeds
- Sunflower seeds
- Walnuts

SWEETENERS

- Erythritol granules
- Stevia powder
- Xylitol granules

VEGETABLES

- All green leafy vegetables (spinach, cabbage, lettuces etc)
- Any other vegetables which are grown above the ground (except butternut)
- Artichoke hearts
- Asparagus
- Aubergines
- Avocados
- Broccoli
- Brussels sprouts
- Cabbage
- Cauliflower
- Celery
- Courgettes
- Leeks
- Mushrooms
- Olives
- Onions
- Peppers
- Pumpkin
- Radishes
- Sauerkraut
- Spring onions
- Tomatoes

Orange List

Chart your carbohydrates without getting obsessive and still obtain an excellent outcome. If you are endeavoring to go into ketosis, this list will assist you to stay under a total of 50g carbs for the day. These are all net carbs and they are all 23 to 25g per indicated amount. Ingredients are all fresh, unless otherwise indicated.

FRUITS

- Apples 1.5
- Bananas 1 small
- Blackberries 3.5 C
- Blueberries 1.5 C
- Cherries (sweet) 1 C
- Clementine's 3
- Figs 3 small
- Gooseberries 1.5 C
- Grapes (green) less than 1 C
- Guavas 2
- Kiwi fruits 3
- Litchis 18
- Mangos, sliced, under 1 C

- Nectarines 2
- Oranges 2
- Pawpaw 1
- Peaches 2
- Pears (Bartlett) 1
- Pineapple, sliced, 1 C
- Plums 4
- Pomegranate ½
- Prickly pears 4
- Quinces 2
- Raspberries 2 C
- Strawberries 25
- Watermelon 2 C

NUTS

- Cashews, raw, 6 T
- Chestnuts, raw, 1 C

SWEETENERS

- Honey 1 t

VEGETABLES

- Butternut 1.5 C
- Carrots 5

- Sweet potato 0.5 C

KEY

C = cups per day

T = tablespoons per day

t = teaspoons per day

g = grams per day

For example 1.5 apples are all the carbs you can have off the orange list for the day (if you want to go into ketosis and make sure you are under 50g total carbs for the day).

Red List

Red will contain all the foods to avoid, as they will be either toxic (e.g. seed oils, soya) or high-carbohydrate foods (e.g. potatoes, rice).

We strongly suggest you avoid all the items on this list, or, at best, eat them very occasionally and restrict the amount when you do. They will do nothing to help you in your attempt to reach your goal.

BAKED GOODS

- All flours from grains - wheat flour, corn flour, rye flour, barley flour, pea flour, rice flour etc
- All forms of bread
- All grains - wheat, oats, barley, rye, amaranth, quinoa, teff etc
- Beans (dried)
- "Breaded" or battered foods
- Brans
- Breakfast cereals, muesli, granola of any kind
- Buckwheat
- Cakes, biscuits, confectionery
- Corn products - popcorn, polenta, corn thins, maize
- Couscous
- Crackers, cracker bread
- Millet
- Pasta, noodles
- Rice
- Rice cakes
- Sorghum
- Spelt
- Thickening agents such as gravy powder, maize starch or stock cubes

DAIRY / DAIRY-RELATED

- Cheese spreads, commercial spreads
- Coffee creamers
- Commercial almond milk
- Condensed milk
- Fat-free anything
- Ice cream
- Puddings
- Reduced-fat cow's milk
- Rice milk
- Soy milk

FATS

- All seed oils (safflower, sunflower, canola, grapeseed, cottonseed, corn)
- Chocolate
- Commercial sauces, marinades, and salad dressings
- Hydrogenated or partially hydrogenated oils including margarine, vegetable oils, vegetable fats

BEVERAGES

- Beer, cider
- Fizzy drinks (sodas) of any description other than carbonated water
- Lite, zero, diet drinks of any description

Ketogenic Diet Foods and their Macros

Protein Source				
	Fats (g)	Net Carbs (g)	Protein (g)	Calories
1 oz. beef sirloin (broiled)	4	0	7.7	69
1 oz. ground beef, 30% fat (broiled)	5.1	0	7.1	77
1 oz. chicken, white meat	1.3	0	8.8	49
1 egg (large)	4.8	0.4	6.3	72
1 slice bacon (baked)	3.5	0	2.9	44
1 oz. smoked ham	2.6	0	6.4	50
1 oz. beef hotdog	8.5	0.5	3.1	92
1 oz. pork chop (broiled)	4.1	0	6.7	65
1 oz. pork ribs (roasted)	8.3	0	6.2	102
1 oz. lamb chop (broiled)	3.9	0	7.3	67
1 oz. tuna (cooked)	1.8	0	8.5	52
1 oz. salmon (raw)	1.8	0	5.6	40
1 oz. shrimp (cooked)	0.1	0	6.8	28

Vegetables				
	Fats (g)	Net Carbs (g)	Protein (g)	Calories
1 oz. spinach (raw)	0.1	0.4	0.8	7
1 oz. romaine lettuce	0.1	0.3	0.4	5
1 oz. broccoli (cooked)	0.1	1.1	0.7	10
1 oz. cauliflower (cooked	0.1	0.5	0.5	7
1 oz. celery (raw)	0	0.3	0.7	5
1 oz. cucumber (raw)	0	1	0.2	4
1 oz. green beans (cooked)	0.1	1.3	0.5	10
1 oz. snow peas (cooked)	0	2.8	1.5	24
1 oz. tomato (raw)	0	0.8	0.3	5
1 oz. butternut squash (baked)	0	2.1	0.3	11
1 oz. green bell pepper	0	0.8	0.2	6
1 clove of garlic	0	1	0.2	4
1 oz. white onion (raw)	0	2.1	0.3	11
1 oz. green onion (raw)	0	1.3	0.5	9
1 oz. avocado	4.4	0.6	0.6	47
1 oz. button mushrooms (raw)	0.2	0.6	0.9	6

Dairy Products				
	Fats (g)	Net Carbs (g)	Protein (g)	Calories
1 oz. whole milk	1	1.5	1	19
1 oz. heavy cream	11	0.8	0.6	103
1 oz. half and half cream	3.5	1.3	0.9	39
1 oz. full-fat sour cream	5.6	0.8	0.6	55
1 oz. whole buttermilk	0.9	1.4	0.9	18
1 oz. cheddar cheese	9.4	0.4	7.1	114
1 oz. whole-milk mozzarella	6.3	0.6	6.3	85
1 oz. parmesan	7.3	0.9	10.1	111
1 oz. Swiss cheese	7.9	1.5	7.6	108
1 oz. mascarpone	13	1	1	130
1 oz. cream cheese	9.7	1.1	1.7	97
1 oz. feta cheese	6	1.2	4	75

Nuts and Seeds			
	Fats (g)	Net Carbs (g)	Protein (g)	Calories
---	---	---	---	---
1 oz. almonds (raw)	15	3	6	170
1 oz. cashew nuts (raw)	13	7	5	160
1 oz. hazelnuts (raw)	17	2	4	176
1 oz. walnuts (raw)	18	2	4	185
1 oz. pistachios (raw)	13	5	6	158
1 oz. pumpkin seeds (raw)	14	1	8	159
1 oz. flax seeds (raw)	10	0	7	131
1 oz. chia seeds (raw)	100	0	7	160
1 oz. sesame seeds (raw)	14	4	5	160

Chapter 3

Creating Your Own Meal Plan

Remember that in order to lose weight on the Ketogenic Diet, you have to let your body enter into the metabolic state of ketosis. Without this, your body will still continue to burn glucose as fuel and would store as fat any excess sugar that isn't used as fuel. In order for you to enter ketosis, you have to decrease your consumption of carbs, increase your intake of fat, and moderately eat protein.

As you know, the foods you eat are key to reset your body and shift you into a different metabolic state. This is why it is very important that you create your own meal plan so that you are sure that everything you eat will not disrupt your metabolism's state of ketosis. My advice is that you *determine the macros that you need to consume through the use of this keto calculator* so that you can achieve weight loss through the diet.

After you have identified the number of grams of macronutrients(carbs, protein & fat) that you should consume daily for your body type, stick with this number when you create your meal plan.

For example, John, who is an average 6-foot tall male who weighs 190 lbs. (86.2 kg) and lives a sedentary lifestyle. According to the keto calculator, in order for John to lose weight and enter ketosis, he must maintain a daily diet of 1654 kcal made with 25g carbs (6%), 91g protein (22%), and 132g fat (72%).

With these numbers— 1654 calories, 25g net carbs, 91g protein, and 132g fat, John should create a meal plan to help him achieve this.

I've provided you with a meal plan in the next chapter of this book that you can use in the early weeks of your Ketogenic Diet, or you can also create a meal plan of your own using the following tips:

Helpful Tips for the Ketogenic Diet

Learn to Count Your Net Carbs— As you now know, the key to entering a state of ketosis is to limit your carbs to 20-50 grams (net carbs) every day. One of the useful tools to help you monitor this is through the use of an app called MyFitnessPal (I encourage you to download this on your device!). With this app, you can easily log your foods which can help you monitor the foods you consume.

Although this app doesn't provide you with your consumption of net carbs, it will provide you with the fiber and carbs that you have consumed. To get your net carbs, just simply subtract the fiber from the carbs you consumed.

Beware of Hidden Carbs— It will be very easy for you to avoid foods such as pasta and bread, because you know that they contain loads of carbs. However, what most people fail to do is to also count the carbs that are "hidden" in foods such as baked beans, salad dressing, and tomato sauce which all have carbs in them! So make sure to read labels and count all carbs to stick to the 20-50 grams daily and achieve ketosis.

Choose the Right Foods— Even if the Ketogenic Diet is a low-carb high-fat diet, this doesn't give you the liberty to consume as much fat as you can. Choosing the right fats (the saturated kind) is key. Stay away from carbs such as pasta, bread, rice and sugar completely. It's just not worth risking it. The 20-50 grams of carbs that you're allowed to consume should be made of nutrient dense vegetables that also have carbs in them.

Limit Your Consumption of Fruit— We all know that fruits have loads of vitaminutes, fiber, and other nutrients that are good for the body. However, if you want to reset your metabolism and allow it to use fat as fuel instead of using glucose, then you must limit your consumption of fruit to a minimum. That's because all fruits are high in fructose (a type of sugar), which causes your insulin levels to spike. When that happens, the fats cells in your body are locked and your body will use glucose as energy.

Remember that on the Ketogenic Diet, you are only allowed to have 25-50 grams of net carbs a day. A medium-sized banana already amounts to 24g net carbs, which means, you almost have already consumed all your carbs for the day in just eating a banana. If you still want to consume fruits, you can stick with a cup of mixed berries that has 5g net carbs, but this is not recommended to be consumed daily.

Spend More Time in the Kitchen— For you to achieve ketosis, it is vital that you watch over the foods you eat. That's why it is advisable foryou to prepare your own meals and avoid eating out too much. Yes, you will have to sacrifice a bit of your time in preparing your meals, but this assures you that you're only consuming what is approved in the Ketogenic Diet.

4 Week Keto Meal Plan

Meal Plan – Week One			
	Monday	**Tuesday**	**Wednesday**
Breakfast	Red Pepper, Mozzarella and Bacon Frittata	Breakfast Quiche	Mahón Kale Sausage Omelet Pie
Lunch	Asian Grilled Chicken	Creamy Haddock	Cheesy Crust Pizza
Dinner	Chorizo Stuffed Bell Peppers	Italian Gnocchi Soup	Bouillabaisse Fish Stew
Thursday	**Friday**	**Saturday**	**Sunday**
Hot n' Spicy Scramble	Breakfast Bread Pudding	Chia Flour Pancakes	Keto Baked Pancetta and Eggs
Rosemary, Chicken Sausage Pies	Chorizo Stuffed Bell Peppers	Lime Avocado Salmon	Meaty Bagels
Stir Fried Beef	Spicy Bacon-Wrapped Dogs	Monterey Jack Steak	Balsamic Pork

Meal Plan – Week Two			
	Monday	**Tuesday**	**Wednesday**
Breakfast	Keto French Almond Toast	Quick Coconut Berry Pancakes	Keto Pork and Sage Breakfast Burgers
Lunch	Savoury Mince	Baked Creamy Cauliflower-Broccoli Chicken	Leftover Meat Salad
Dinner	Mediterranean Chicken	Pulled Pork Shoulder	Keto Friendly Sushi
Thursday	**Friday**	**Saturday**	**Sunday**
Millet Gingerbread Mash	Egg Whites and Spinach Omelet	Hemp Muffins with Walnuts	Baked Ham and Kale Scrambled Eggs
Shrimp & Avocado Salad	Spring Roll in a Bowl	Cheese Steak Salad	Turkey Meatballs
Chicken Parmesan	Baked Pork Chops in Sweet-Sour Marinade	Salmon Burgers	Chicken Satay

Meal Plan – Week Three			
	Monday	**Tuesday**	**Wednesday**
Breakfast	Fast Protein and Peanut-Butter Pancakes	Vesuvius Scrambled Eggs with Provolone	Keto Oatmeal
Lunch	Chicken Pot Pie	Mackerel Salad	Spicy Mexican Meatballs
Dinner	Baked Glazed Salmon	Zesty Herbed Chicken	Sweet and Sour Snapper
Thursday	**Friday**	**Saturday**	**Sunday**
Crimini Mushroom with Boiled Eggs Breakfast	Anchovy, Spinach and Asparagus Omelet	Guacamole Bacon and Eggs Breakfast	Keto Bilberry Coconut Mush
Salmon Salad in Avo Cups	Creamy Chicken Salad	Bell Peppers Stuffed	Cheeseburger Casserole
Pordenone Cauliflower Lasagna	Lemon Mustard Pork Loin	Seared Ribeye Steak	Macadamia Crusted Lamb Chops

Meal Plan – Week Four			
	Monday	**Tuesday**	**Wednesday**
Breakfast	Chocó Mocha Chia Porridge	Keto Pancakes and Syrup	Mediterranean Egg Scramble
Lunch	Chicken and Broccoli filled Zucchini	Cheesy Bacon Spinach Log	Meatballs in Coconut Broth
Dinner	Lamb Curry & Spinach	Slow-Cooker Stroganoff	Bolognese Squash Spaghetti
Thursday	**Friday**	**Saturday**	**Sunday**
Chorizo Breakfast Peppers	Autumn Keto Pumpkin Bread	Chicharrones con Huevos (Pork Rind and Eggs)	Baked Buckwheat Pancakes with Hazelnuts
Glazed Sesame Ginger Salmon	Spicy Chicken Thighs	Blackberry and Grilled Chicken Salad	Sunday's Best Roast Beef
Lamb Cutlets with Garlic Sauce	Beanless Chili con Carne	Tomato Bredie	Pad Thai

Chapter 4: Breakfasts

"Cooking With Love Provides Food for the Soul"

Keto Pancakes and Syrup

(Total Time: 30 MIN| Serve: 5)

Ingredients:

For Syrup:
2 tbsp maple syrup, sugar-free
½ cup Sukrin fiber syrup

For Pancakes:
4 eggs, large
2 Tbsp erythritol
½ tsp baking soda
3/4 cup nut butter of your choice
1/3 cup coconut milk
2 tbsp ghee
1 tsp cinnamon

Directions:

1. Add maple syrup and sukrin fiber syrup into a jar or small bowl and use a spoon to stir until combined. Cover jar and put aside until needed.
2. Put eggs, erythritol, baking soda, coconut milk, nut butter and cinnamon powder in a food processor and pulse until blended.
3. Heat ghee in a non-stick skillet and use about a ¼ cup per pancake. Cook until pancake sets, then flip and finish cooking; place on a plate.
4. Repeat with remaining batter and plate.
5. Top with syrup and serve.

(Calories 401 | Total Fats 32.5g | Net Carbs: 3.6g | Protein 12.8g)

Bacon Avocado Breakfast Muffins

(Total Time: 41 MIN| Serve: 16)

Ingredients:

½ cup almond flour
1 ½ Tbsp psyllium husk powder
4.5 oz Colby jack cheese
1 tsp baking powder
1 tsp garlic, diced
1 tsp chives, dried
3 stalks spring onions
1 tsp cilantro, dried
¼ tsp red chili flakes
Salt and pepper
1 ½ Tbsp lemon juice
5 eggs
¼ cup flaxseed meal
1 ½ cup coconut milk, from box
5 slices bacon, cubed
2 avocados, cubed
2 Tbsp butter, organic

Directions:

1. Add flour, spices, lemon juice, eggs, flaxseed meal and coconut milk to a bowl. Mix together until thoroughly combined.
2. Heat a skillet and cook bacon cubes until crispy then add the butter and avocado.
3. Add the bacon and avocado mixture to batter and mix together.
4. Set oven to 350 F and grease cupcake molds.
5. Add batter to molds and bake for 26 minutes. Take from oven and cool before removing from mold.
6. Serve. Store leftovers in the fridge.

(Calories 163 | Total Fats 14.1g | Net Carbs: 1.5g | Protein 6.1g)

Orange Cinnamon Scones

(Total Time: 30 MIN| Serve: 8)

Ingredients:

1 tbsp golden flax seed

1 ½ tsp cinnamon

½ tsp salt

7 Tbsp + 1 Tbsp coconut flour

½ tsp baking powder

Zest from one orange

¼ cup butter, unsalted, cubed

¼ cup erythritol

¼ tsp stevia

2 eggs

2 Tbsp maple syrup

½ tsp xanthan gum

1/3 cup heavy cream

1 tsp vanilla

For Icing:

20 drops stevia

1 Tbsp orange juice

¼ cup coconut butter

Directions:

1. Set oven to 400 F.
2. Place all dry ingredients in a bowl except xanthan and 1 Tbsp coconut flour. Add butter to dry mixture and stir to combine.
3. Combine sweetener and eggs until thoroughly mixed and light in color. Put in maple syrup, remaining flour, xanthan gum, heavy cream and vanilla; mix until combined and thick.
4. Add wet mixture to dry, reserving 2 Tbsp of liquids, mix together and add cinnamon and use hands to form mixture into dough. Shape into a flat square and slice into 8 even pieces.
5. Place onto a lined baking sheet and use reserved liquid to brush the top of scones.
6. Bake for 15 minutes, remove from oven and cool.
7. Prepare icing and drizzle over scones before serving.

(Calories 232 | Total Fats 20g | Net Carbs: 3.3g | Protein 3.3g)

Red Pepper, Mozzarella and Bacon Frittata

(Total Time: 35 MIN| **Serve: 6**)

Ingredients:

1 tbsp olive oil
7 slices bacon
1 red bell pepper, chopped
¼ cup heavy cream
¼ cup parmesan cheese, grated
9 eggs
Salt and pepper
2 Tbsp parsley, chopped
4 cups Bella mushrooms, large
½ cup basil, chopped
4 oz mozzarella cheese, cubed
2 oz goat cheese, chopped

Directions:

1. Set oven to 350 F.
2. Heat olive oil in a skillet then add bacon and cook for 5 minutes until browned.
3. Add red pepper and cook for 2 minutes until soft. While pepper cooks, add cream, parmesan cheese, eggs, parsley, salt, and pepper to a bowl and whisk to combine.
4. Add mushrooms to pot, stir and cook for 5 minutes until soaked in fat. Add basil, cook for 1 minute then add mozzarella.
5. Add in egg mixture and use a spoon to move ingredients around so that the egg gets on the bottom of the pan.
6. Top with goat cheese and place in oven for 8 minutes, then broil for 6 minutes.
7. Use a knife to pry frittata edges from pan and place on a plate and slice.

(Calories 408 | Total Fats 31.2g | Net Carbs: 2.4g | Protein 19.2g)

Cheese and Sausage Pies

(Total Time: 40 MIN| Serve: 2)

Ingredients:

1 ½ pieces chicken sausage
½ tsp rosemary
¼ tsp baking soda
¼ cup coconut flour
¼ tsp cayenne pepper
1/8 tsp salt
5 egg yolks
2 tsp lemon juice
¼ cup coconut oil
2 Tbsp coconut milk
¾ cheddar cheese, grated

Directions:

1. Set oven to 350 F.
2. Chop sausage, heat skillet and cook sausage. While sausages cook, combine all dry ingredients in a bowl. In another bowl, combine egg yolks, lemon juice, oil and coconut milk. Add liquids to dry mixture and add ½ cup of cheese; fold to combine and put into 2 ramekins.
3. Add cooked sausages to the batter and use a spoon to push into the mixture.
4. Bake for 25 minutes until golden on top. Top with leftover cheese and broil for 4 minutes.
5. Serve warm.

(Calories 711 | Total Fats 65.3g | Net Carbs: 5.8g | Protein 34.3g)

Breakfast Quiche

(Total Time: 30 MIN| **Serve:** 2)

Ingredients:

3 tbsp coconut oil
5 eggs
8 slices bacon, cooked and chopped
½ cup cream
2 cups baby spinach, roughly chopped
1 cup red pepper, chopped
1 cup yellow onion, chopped
2 cloves garlic, minced
1 cup mushrooms, chopped
1 cup cheddar cheese, grated
Salt

Directions:

1. Preheat oven to 375 F.
2. In a large bowl, mix all vegetables including the mushrooms together.
3. In another small bowl, whisk the 5 eggs with the cream.
4. Carefully scoop the veggie mixture into a muffin pan coated with cooking spray, top with egg and cheese filling up to ¾ of the muffin tins. Sprinkle with chopped bacon on top.
5. Place in the oven to bake for 15 minutes, or until the top of the quiches are firm.
6. Let them cool for a few minutes before serving.

(Calories 210 | Total Fats 13g | Net Carbs: 5g | Protein 6g)

Chicharrones con Huevos (Pork Rind and Eggs)

(Total Time: 30 MIN| Serve: 3)

Ingredients:

4 slices bacon
1.5 oz pork rinds
1 avocado, cubed
¼ cup onion, chopped
1 tomato, chopped
2 jalapeno pepper, seeds removed and chopped
5 eggs
¼ cup cilantro
Salt and pepper

Directions:

1. Heat skillet and cook bacon until slightly crisp. Remove from pot and put aside on paper towels.
2. Add pork rinds to the pot, along with onion, tomatoes and pepper and cook for 3 minutes, until onions are soft and clear.
3. Add cilantro, stir together gently and add eggs. Scramble eggs and then add avocado and fold.
4. Serve.

(Calories 508 | Total Fats 43g | Net Carbs: 12g | Protein 5g)

Raspberry & Cacao Breakfast Bowl

(Total Time: 40 MIN| Serve: 1)

Ingredients:

1 cup almond milk
1 Tbsp cacao powder
3 Tbsp chia seeds
¼ cup raspberries
1 tsp agave or xylitol

Directions:

1. In a small bowl, combine the almond milk and cocoa powder. Stir well.
2. Add the chia seeds to the bowl and let it rest for 5 minutes.
3. Using a fork, fluff the chia and cacao mixture and then place in the fridge to chill for at least 30 minutes.
4. Serve with raspberries and a drizzle of agave on top

(Calories 230 | Total Fats 20g | Net Carbs: 4g | Protein 15g)

Anaheim Pepper Gruyere Waffles

(Total Time: 16 MIN| **S**erve: 2)

Ingredients:

1 small Anaheim pepper
3 eggs
1/4 cup cream cheese
1/4 cup Gruyere cheese
1 Tbsp coconut flour
1 tsp Metamucil powder
1 tsp baking powder
Salt and pepper to taste

Directions:

1. In a blender, mix together all ingredients, except for the Gruyere cheese and Anaheim pepper. Once the ingredients are mixed well, add cheese and pepper. Blend well until all ingredients are mixed well.
2. Heat your waffle iron; pour on the waffle mixture and cook 5-6 minutes. Serve hot.

(Calories 223.55 | Total Fats 17g | Net Carbs: 5.50g | Protein 11g)

Nutty Cocoa Cereal

(Total Time: 12 MIN| Serve: 2)

Ingredients:

3 tsp organic butter
¾ cup toasted walnuts, roughly chopped
¾ cup toasted macadamia nuts, roughly chopped
½ cup coconut shreds, unsweetened
½ Tbsp stevia (optional)
2 cups almond milk
1/8 tsp salt

Directions:

1. Melt the butter in a pot over the medium heat. Add the toasted nuts to the pot and stir for 2 minutes.
2. Add the shredded coconut into the pot and continue stirring to make sure to not burn the ingredients.
3. Drizzle with stevia (if using) and then pour the milk into the pot. Add salt. Stir again and turn the heat off.
4. Allow resting for 10 minutes to allow the ingredients to soak in the milk before serving.

(Calories 515 | Total Fats 50.3g | Net Carbs: 14.4g | Protein 6.5g)

Breakfast Tacos

(Total Time: 25 MIN| **Serve:** 3)

Ingredients:

3 strips bacon
1 cup mozzarella cheese, shredded
2 Tbsp butter
6 eggs
Salt and pepper
½ avocado, cubed
1 oz cheddar cheese, shredded

Directions:

1. Cook bacon until crisp, put aside until needed.
2. Heat a non-stick pan and place 1/3 cup mozzarella into the pan and cook for 3 minutes until browned around the edges. Place a wooden spoon in a bowl or pot and use tongs to lift cheese 'taco from the pot. Repeat with leftover cheese.
3. Melt butter in a skillet and scramble eggs; use pepper and salt to season.
4. Spoon eggs into hardened shells and top with avocado and bacon.
5. Top with cheddar and serve.

(Calories 443 | Total Fats 36.2g | Net Carbs: 3g | Protein 25.7g)

Cheesy Bacon and Chive Omelet

(Total Time: 30 MIN| Serve: 1)

Ingredients:

2 eggs, large
Salt and pepper
1 tsp bacon fat
1 oz cheddar cheese
2 slices bacon, cooked
2 stalks chives

Directions:

1. Beat eggs together and add pepper and salt to taste. Chop chives and shred cheese.
2. Heat skillet and cook bacon fat until hot.
3. Add eggs to pot and top with chives. Cook until edges start to set, then add bacon and cook for 30-60 seconds.
4. Add cheese and a few additional chives. Use a spatula to fold in half. Press to seal and flip over.
5. Serve immediately.

(Calories 463 | Total Fats 39g | Net Carbs: 1g | Protein 24g)

Pizza Waffles

(Total Time: 30 MIN| **Serve**: 2)

Ingredients:

1 Tbsp psyllium husk
1 tsp baking powder
Salt
3 oz cheddar cheese
4 eggs, large
3 Tbsp almond flour
1 Tbsp butter, organic
1 tsp Italian seasoning
4 Tbsp parmesan cheese
½ cup tomato sauce

Directions:

1. Add all ingredients to a bowl, except cheese and tomato sauce. Use mixer or immersion blender to combine until mixture is thick.
2. Heat waffle iron and use mixture to make two waffles.
3. Place waffles onto a lined baking sheet and top with tomato sauce and cheese (divide evenly). Broil for 3 minutes or until cheese melted.
4. Serve.

(Calories 525.5 | Total Fats 41.5g | Net Carbs: 5g | Protein 29g)

Anchovy, Spinach and Asparagus Omelet

(Total Time: 23 MIN| **Serve**: 2)

Ingredients:

2 oz anchovies in olive oil
2 organic eggs
3/4 cup of spinach
4 marinated asparagus
Celtic sea salt
Freshly ground black pepper

Directions:

1. Preheat the oven to 375 F.
2. In the bottom of the baking pan place the anchovies.
3. In a bowl, beat the eggs and pour on top of the fish. Add the spinach and the chopped asparagus on top.
4. Season with salt and pepper to taste.
5. Bake in preheated oven for about 10 minutes.
6. Serve hot.

(Calories 83 | Total Fats 4.91g | Net Carbs: 2.28g | Protein 7.5g)

Autumn Keto Pumpkin Bread

(Total Time: 1 HR 30 MIN| Serve: 2)

Ingredients:

3 egg whites
1/2 cup coconut milk
1 1/2 cup almond flour
1/2 cup pumpkin puree
2 tsp baking powder
1 1/2 tsp Pumpkin pie spice
1/2 tsp Kosher Salt
Coconut oil for greasing

Directions:

1. Preheat your oven to 350F. Grease a standard bread loaf pan with melted coconut oil.
2. Sift all dry ingredients into a large bowl.
3. In another bowl, add pumpkin puree and coconut milk and mix well. In a separate bowl, beat the egg whites. Fold in egg whites and gently fold into the dough.
4. Spread the dough into the prepared bread pan.
5. Bake the bread for 75 minutes. Once ready, remove bread from the oven and let cool.
6. Slice and serve.

(Calories 197 | Total Fats 16g | Net Carbs: 8.18g | Protein 7.2g)

Keto Oatmeal

(Total Time: 20 MIN| **Serve:** 5)

Ingredients:

1/3 cup almonds, flaked
1/3 cup unsweetened coconut flakes
¼ cup chia seeds
2 Tbsp erythritol
¼ cup coconut, shredded, unsweetened
1 cup almond milk
1 tsp vanilla, sugar-free
10 drops stevia extract
½ cup heavy whipping cream, whipped

Directions:

1. Place almonds and coconut flakes in a pot and toast for 3 minutes until fragrant.
2. Place toasted ingredients into a bowl along with chia seeds, erythritol, and shredded coconut; mix together to combine.
3. Top with milk and stir. You can use hot or cold milk based on your preference.
4. Add vanilla and stevia, stir and set aside for 5-10 minutes.
5. Serve topped with whipped cream.

(Calories 277 | Total Fats 25.6g | Net Carbs: 16.4g | Protein 5.5g)

Batter Coated Cheddar Cheese

(Total Time: 23 MIN| Serve: 1)

Ingredients:

1 large egg
2 slices Cheddar cheese
1 tsp ground walnuts
1 tsp ground flaxseed
2 tsp almond flour
1 tsp hemp seeds
1 Tbsp olive oil
Salt and pepper to taste

Directions:

1. In a small bowl, whisk an egg together with the salt and pepper.
2. Heat a tbsp of olive oil in a frying pan, on medium heat.
3. In a separate bowl, mix the ground flaxseed with the ground walnuts, hemp seeds, and the almond flour.
4. Coat the cheddar slices with the egg mixture, then roll in the dry mixture and fry cheese for about 3 minutes on each side. Serve hot.

(Calories 509 | Total Fats 16g | Net Carbs: 2g | Protein 21g)

Mahón Kale Sausage Omelet Pie

(Total Time: 40 MIN| **Serve: 8**)

Ingredients:

3 chicken sausages
2 1/2 cups mushrooms, chopped
3 cups fresh spinach
10 eggs
1/2 tsp black pepper and celery seed
2 tsp hot sauce
1 Tbsp garlic powder
Salt and pepper to taste
1 1/2 cups Mahón cheese (or Cheddar)

Directions:

1. Preheat oven to 400 F.
2. Chop up the mushroom and chicken sausage thin and place them in a cast iron skillet. Cook on a medium-high heat for 2-3 minutes.
3. While the sausages are cooking, chopped spinach, then add spinach and mushrooms to the skillet.
4. In a meanwhile, in a bowl mix eggs with black pepper and celery seed, spices, and hot sauce. Scramble all mixture well.
5. Mix your spinach, mushrooms, and sausages so that the spinach can wilt completely. Season with salt and pepper to taste.
6. Finally, add the cheese to the top.
7. Pour eggs over the mixture and combine well.
8. Stir the mixture for a few seconds, and then place your skillet in the oven. Bake for 10-12 minutes, and then broil the top for 4 minutes.
9. Let cool for a while, cut into 8 slices and serve hot.

(Calories 266 | Total Fats 17g | Net Carbs: 7g | Protein 19g)

Monterey Bacon-Scallions Omelet

(Total Time: 30 MIN| **Serve:** 2)

Ingredients:

2 eggs
2 slices cooked bacon
1/4 cup scallions, chopped
1/4 cup Monterey Jack cheese
Salt and pepper to taste
1 tsp lard

Directions:

1. In a frying pan heat lard in on medium-low heat. Add the eggs, scallions and salt and pepper to taste.
2. Cook for 1-2 minutes; add the bacon and sauté 30 - 45 seconds longer. Turn the heat off on the stove.
3. On top of the bacon place a cheese. Then, take two edges of the omelet and fold them onto the cheese. Hold the edges there for a moment as the cheese has to partially melt. Do the same with the other egg and let cook in a warm pan for a while.
4. Serve hot.

(Calories 321 | Total Fats 28g | Net Carbs: 1.62g | Protein 14g)

Smoked Turkey Bacon and Avocado Muffins

(Total Time: 45 MIN| Serve: 16)

Ingredients:

6 slices smoked turkey bacon
2 Tbsp butter
3 spring onions
1/2 cup cheddar cheese
1 tsp baking powder
1 1/2 cups coconut milk
5 eggs
1 1/2 Tbsp Metamucil powder
1/2 cup almond flour
1/4 cup flaxseed
1 tsp minced garlic
2 tsp dried parsley
1/4 tsp red chili powder
1 1/2 Tbsp lemon juice
Salt and pepper to taste
2 medium avocados

Directions:

1. Preheat oven to 350 F.
2. In a frying pan over medium-low heat, cook the bacon with the butter until crisp. Add the spring onions, cheese, and baking powder.
3. In a bowl, mix together coconut milk, eggs, Metamucil powder, almond flour, flax, spices and lemon juice. Switch off the heat and let cool. Then, crumble the bacon and add all of the fat to the egg mixture.
4. Clean and chop avocado and fold into the mixture.
5. Measure out batter into a cupcake tray that's been sprayed or greased with nonstick spray and bake for 25-26 minutes.
6. Once ready, let cool and serve hot or cold.

(Calories 184 | Total Fats 16g | Net Carbs: 5.51g | Protein 5.89g)

Hot n' Spicy Scramble

(Total Time: 25 MIN| **Serve:** 4)

Ingredients:

1 green bell pepper, chopped
1 onion, chopped
1 cup cooked ham, diced
1 cup pepper jack cheese, shredded
8 organic eggs
½ tsp chili powder
1 tsp Sriracha sauce
¼ cup coconut milk
Salt and pepper to taste
2 tbsp ghee

Directions:

1. Heat the ghee in a non-stick pan over medium fire.
2. Add the onions and bell pepper to the pan and sauté for 5 minutes.
3. Season with salt and pepper and add the diced ham into the pan.
4. Meanwhile, in a large bowl, whisk together the eggs, chili powder, Sriracha sauce, and coconut milk.
5. Gradually add the shredded cheese into the bowl with eggs. Set aside.
6. Reduce the heat to low and then pour the egg mixture into the pan with the bell peppers and cook for 2 minutes.
7. Flip and then cook again until the eggs are done.
8. Serve.

(Calories 545 | Total Fats 53.6g | Net Carbs: 10g | Protein 35g)

Chorizo Breakfast Peppers

(Total Time: 25 MIN| Serve: 2)

Ingredients:

½ tbsp ghee
1 onion, chopped
2 cloves of garlic
6 organic eggs
¼ cup almond milk, unsweetened
1 cup cheddar cheese, shredded
Salt and pepper to taste
3 large bell peppers, cut in half, core and seeds removed
½ lb. spicy chorizo sausage, crumbled

Directions:

1. Set oven to 350 F.
2. Heat the ghee in a non-stick pan over medium heat and cook the chorizo crumbles. Set aside
3. Using the same pan, add the onions and garlic and sauté for a few minutes. Turn off the heat and set aside.
4. In a bowl, stir together the eggs, milk, cheddar, and season with salt and pepper.
5. Add the chorizo into the bowl with the eggs and stir well.
6. Place the bell pepper halves in an oven-safe dish filled with a ¼ inch of water.
7. Scoop the chorizo and egg mixture into the bell peppers and place the dish into the oven to bake for 35 minutes.
8. Serve warm.

(Calories 631 | Total Fats 46g | Net Carbs: 13g | Protein 44g)

Breakfast Bread Pudding

(Total Time: 30 MIN| Serve: 2)

Ingredients:

4 slices of the Protein Loaded bread, chopped into small bites
2 organic eggs
2 tbsp heavy cream
2 tbsp stevia
1 tsp cinnamon, ground
1 Tbsp organic butter

Directions:

1. Set oven to 350 F.
2. In a bowl whisk the eggs with heavy cream and stevia.
3. Place the chopped bread into an oven-safe dish and pour over the egg mixture. Sprinkle with cinnamon.
4. Bake in the oven for 15 minutes or until the pudding has set.
5. Allow to cool before serving warm.

(Calories 278 | Total Fats 19.5g | Net Carbs: 4.1g | Protein 22.4g)

Creamy Chocó & Avocado Mousse

(Total Time: 50 MIN| **Serve:** 2)

Ingredients:

2 ripe avocados
1/3 cup cocoa powder
½ tsp chia seeds
1 tsp vanilla extract
10 drops Stevie
3 Tbsp coconut oil

Directions:

1. Place all the ingredients in a blender and blend until smooth.
2. Pour the mixture into a bowl or separate glass bowls, and place in the fridge to chill for 40 minutes or more.
3. Serve chilled.

(Calories 462 | Total Fats 46g | Net Carbs: 15g | Protein 6g)

Sour Cream Cheese Pancakes

(Total Time: 30 MIN| Serve: 2)

Ingredients:

2 eggs
1/4 cup cream cheese
1 Tbsp coconut flour
1 tsp ground ginger
1/2 cup liquid Stevia
Coconut oil
Sugar-free maple syrup

Directions:

1. In a deep bowl, beat together all of the ingredients until smooth.
2. Heat up a frying skillet with oil on medium-high. Ladle the batter into hot oil in tablespoon size quantities.
3. Cook on one side and then flip. Top with a sugar-free maple syrup and serve.

(Calories 170 | Total Fats 13g | Net Carbs: 4g | Protein 6.90g)

Vesuvius Scrambled Eggs with Provolone

(Total Time: 15 MIN| Serve: 2)

Ingredients:

2 large eggs
3/4 cup Provolone cheese
1.76 oz. air-dried salami
1 tsp fresh rosemary (chopped)
1 Tbsp olive oil
Salt and pepper to taste

Directions:

1. In a small pan with olive oil, fry the chopped salami.
2. In the meantime, in a small bowl, whisk the eggs, then add the salt, pepper and fresh rosemary.
3. Add in the provolone cheese and mix well with a fork.
4. Pour the egg mixture into the pan with salami and cook for about 5 minutes. Serve hot.

(Calories 396 | Total Fats 32.4g | Net Carbs: 2.8g | Protein 26.1g)

Adorable Pumpkin Flaxseed Muffins

(Total Time: 25 MIN| **Serve:** 2)

Ingredients:

1 egg
1 1/4 cups flax seeds (ground)
1 cup pumpkin puree
1 Tbsp pumpkin pie spice
2 Tbsp coconut oil
1/2 cup sweetener of your choice
1 tsp baking powder
2 tsp cinnamon
1/2 tsp apple cider vinegar
1/2 tsp vanilla extract
Salt to taste
Stiffly whipped cream to decorate

Directions:

1. Preheat your oven to 360 F.
2. First, grind the flaxseeds for several seconds.
3. Put together all the dry ingredients and stir.
4. Then, add your pumpkin puree and mix to combine.
5. Add the vanilla extract and the pumpkin spice.
6. Add in coconut oil, egg and apple vinegar. Add sweetener of your choice and stir again.
7. Add a heaped tbsp of batter to each lined muffin or cupcake pan and top with some pumpkin seeds.
8. Bake for about 18 - 20 minutes. Take out of the oven, extract from pan and cool slightly on a rack
9. Pipe stiffly beaten cream on top and serve warm.

(Calories 43| Total Fats 5.34g | Net Carbs: 3g | Protein 1g)

Baked Ham and Kale Scrambled Eggs

(Total Time: 40 MIN| **Serve:** 2)

Ingredients:

5 ounces ham diced
2 medium eggs
1 green onion, finely chopped
1/2 cups kale leaves, chopped
1 garlic clove, crushed
1 green chili, finely chopped
4 ready-roasted peppers
Pinch cayenne pepper
1 Tbsp olive oil
1/2 cup water

Directions:

1. Heat oven to 360 F.
2. Heat the oil in a small ovenproof frying pan. Add green onion and cook for 4-5 minutes until softened.
3. Stir in the garlic and chili, and cook for a couple minutes more.
4. Add the 1/2 cup water. Season well and stir in the ready-roasted peppers and ham. Bring to a simmer and cook for 10 minutes.
5. Add the kale, stirring through to wilt.
6. In a small bowl, beat the eggs with a pinch of cayenne and pour in frying pan together with other ingredients.
7. Transfer the frying pan to the oven and bake for 10 minutes.
8. Serve hot.

(Calories 251| Total Fats 15.74g | Net Carbs: 3.8g | Protein 22g)

Bell Pepper and Ham Omelet

(Total Time: 30 MIN| Serve: 2)

Ingredients:

4 large eggs
1 cup green pepper, chopped
1/4 lb ham, cooked and diced
1 green onion, diced
1 tsp coconut oil
Salt and freshly ground pepper to taste

Directions:

1. Wash and chop vegetables. Set aside.
2. Into a small bowl beat the eggs. Set aside.
3. Heat a non-stick skillet over medium heat and add coconut oil. Pour half of the beaten eggs into the skillet.
4. When the egg has partially set, add half of the vegetables and ham to one-half of the omelet and continue to cook until the egg is almost fully set.
5. Fold the empty half over top of the ham and veggies using a spatula.
6. Cook for 2 minutes more and then Keep warm.
7. Repeat procedure for second serving. Serve hot.

(Calories 225.76 | Total Fats 12g | Net Carbs: 6.8g | Protein 21.88g)

Chia Flour Pancakes

(Total Time: 25 MIN| **Serve:** 6)

Ingredients:

1 cup chia flour
2 tsp sweetener of your choice
1 egg, beaten
1 tbsp coconut butter or oil
1/2 cup coconut milk (canned)

Directions:

1. In a medium bowl, combine the flour and sweetener. Add the egg, milk and coconut butter. Mix well until it makes a smooth batter.
2. Grease a non-stick skillet and heat over medium-high heat. Drop a heaped Tbsp of batter onto the hot surface.
3. When bubbles form on the surface of the scones, use a spatula to turn them and then cook about 2 minutes per side.
4. Serve hot.

(Calories 59 | Total Fats 3.5g | Net Carbs: 4.65g | Protein 2.46g)

Chocó Mocha Chia Porridge

(Total Time: 35 MIN| Serve: 6)

Ingredients:

3 Tbsp chia seeds
1 cup almond milk, unsweetened
2 tsp cocoa powder
1/4 cup raspberries, fresh or frozen
2 Tbsp almonds, ground
Sweetener of your choice

Directions:

1. Mix and stir the almond milk and the cocoa powder together.
2. Add the Chia Seeds into the mixture.
3. Mix well with a fork.
4. Place the mixture in a fridge for 30 minutes.
5. Serve with raspberries and ground almonds on the top (optional)

(Calories 150.15 | Total Fats 9.62g | Net Carbs: 15.2g | Protein 5.47g)

Crimini Mushroom with Boiled Eggs Breakfast

(Total Time: 25 MIN| **Serve:** 6)

Ingredients:

14 crimini mushrooms, finely chopped
8 large eggs, hard-boiled, chopped
6 slices bacon or pancetta
1 spring onion, diced
Salt and ground black pepper to taste

Directions:

1. In a frying pan, cook bacon. Reserve the bacon fat in the pan. Chop up bacon pieces and set aside.
2. In a deep saucepan, hard-boil the eggs. When ready, wash, clean, shell and chop into bite-size pieces.
3. In a frying pan, cook the spring onion with remaining bacon fat over medium-high heat.
4. Add the Crimini mushrooms and sauté another 5-6 minutes.
5. Blend the eggs and bacon and cook together. Adjust salt and ground black pepper to taste.
6. Serve.

(Calories 176.15 | Total Fats 13.38g | Net Carbs: 2.43g | Protein 11.32g)

Egg Whites and Spinach Omelet

(Total Time: 25 MIN| **Serve:** 2)

Ingredients:

5 egg whites
2 Tbsp almond milk
1 zucchini, shredded
1 cup spinach leaves, fresh
2 Tbsp spring onion, chopped
2 cloves garlic
Olive oil
Basil leaves, fresh, chopped
Salt and ground black pepper to taste

Directions:

1. Wash and chop the vegetables
2. In a bowl, beat the egg whites and the almond milk.
3. In a greased frying pan with olive oil, cook the vegetables (spinach, zucchini, and spring onion) just for one to two minutes.
4. Put the vegetables on the side, grease the pan again with olive oil and pour the eggs into it. Cook until the eggs are firm.
5. Add the vegetables on one side and cook for two minutes more. Adjust salt and pepper to taste.
6. Decorate with basil leaves and serve.

(Calories 70.8 | Total Fats 1.56g | Net Carbs: 5.78g | Protein 11.08g)

Fast Protein and Peanut-Butter Pancakes

(Total Time: 15 MIN| Serve: 1)

Ingredients:

1 scoop of low-carb protein powder
2 eggs
2 Tbsp of natural peanut butter
2 Tbsp flaxseed
2 Tbsp water
Olive oil for greasing

Directions:

1. In a bowl, mix protein powder, eggs, peanut butter, water, and flaxseeds.
2. Grease with olive oil and heat a large non-stick frying pan over medium heat.
3. Ladle the batter mixture in small amounts into the pan and cook for 2 minutes per side or until bubbles appear on the surface. Transfer to a plate.
4. Serve hot.

(Calories 406.41 | Total Fats 23.59g | Net Carbs: 13.78g | Protein 17.8g)

Hemp Muffins with Walnuts

(Total Time: 35 MIN| **Serve:** 12)

Ingredients:

2 1/2 cup Hemp flour
1 1/2 cup walnuts, chopped
1/2 cup sweetener of your choice
4 Tbsp extra-virgin olive oil
1 tsp vanilla extract
2 tsp baking powder
1 tsp baking soda

Directions:

1. Preheat oven to 345 F.
2. In a small bowl, whisk olive oil, sweetener of your choice and vanilla.
3. In a separate bowl, combine hemp flour, baking powder, and baking soda. Add in chopped walnuts and toss to coat.
4. Add olive oil mixture to the flour mixture and stir slightly.
5. Spoon a batter into 12 muffin cups, filling 3/4 full.
6. Bake 18 - 20 minutes. Allow to cool 10 minutes in the muffin pan, and then turn out onto a wire rack to cool completely. Serve.

(Calories 301 | Total Fats 17.2g | Net Carbs: 17.8g | Protein 21.5g)

Keto Baked Pancetta and Eggs

(Total Time: 20 MIN| **Serve: 6**)

Ingredients:

6 slices Pancetta, crumbled
8 eggs
3/4 cup Cheddar cheese, grated
3/4 cup heavy cream
Salt and pepper to taste
Olive oil for greasing

Directions:

1. Preheat the oven to 350 F. Grease a big baking dish with olive oil.
2. In a bowl, beat the eggs with shredded Cheddar cheese and cream, and season with salt and pepper to taste.
3. Crumble Pancetta evenly over the egg mixture. Put the baking dish in a preheated oven.
4. Bake for 15 minutes.
5. Serve immediately.

(Calories 295 | Total Fats 24g | Net Carbs: 1.3g | Protein 18.3g)

Keto Bilberry Coconut Mush

(Total Time: 25 MIN| **Serve:** 2)

Ingredients:

1/4 cup coconut flour
1 cup coconut milk
1/4 cup ground flaxseed
1 tsp vanilla extract
1 tsp cinnamon
Liquid sweetener of your choice

Toppings
1 cup bilberries
2 Tbsp shaved coconut
2 Tbsp pumpkin seeds

Directions:

1. In a saucepan, heat the coconut milk. Add in coconut flour, cinnamon and flaxseed and whisk.
2. Add in vanilla extract and liquid sweetener of your choice. Cook for 10 minutes stirring constantly. Remove from heat and let cool for 2-3 minutes.
3. Decorate with fresh bilberries, pumpkin seeds and shaved coconut to taste.

(Calories 445 | Total Fats 22.4g | Net Carbs: 16.4g | Protein 2.86g)

Keto French Almond Toast

(Total Time: 25 MIN| **Serve:** 6)

Ingredients:

4 eggs
1/4 cup coconut milk
2 Tbsp coconut oil, melted
6 slices almond bread
2 tsp sweetener of your choice (optional)
1/2 tsp cinnamon powder
1 tsp organic vanilla extract
Salt and pepper (per taste)

Directions:

1. Whisk coconut milk, sweetener of your choice, eggs, organic vanilla extract, salt, and cinnamon.
2. Soak each slice of almond bread (or any gluten-free vegan Hemp & Seed bread) in egg mixture.
3. In a frying pan, heat the coconut oil over high heat; cook each slice of bread three minutes or until golden. Transfer toast to the plate lined with paper.
4. Serve hot.

(Calories 162.6 | Total Fats 10.2g | Net Carbs: 2.4g | Protein 6.56g)

Pork and Sage Breakfast Burgers

(Total Time: 15 MIN| Serve: 4)

Ingredients:

1 lb ground pork
2 Tbsp fresh sage, chopped
1 tsp garlic powder
1 tsp cayenne pepper
Salt and pepper to taste
2 Tbsp granular sweetener of your choice
Olive oil for greasing

Directions:

1. In a large bowl, combine all ingredients except olive oil. Use hands to mix thoroughly.
2. Form into 8 evenly sized burger patties.
3. Grease your large frying pan with olive oil over medium heat.
4. Add burger pattiesand cook about 3 to 4 minutes per side.
5. Serve and enjoy.

(Calories 302.21 | Total Fats 22.17g | Net Carbs: 0.03g | Protein 19.29g)

Quick Coconut Berry Pancakes

(Total Time: 10 MIN| **Serve:** 2)

Ingredients:

1 Tbsp butter, melted
2 eggs
5 Tbsp full-fat milk
1 Tbsp xylitol
½ tsp salt
2 Tbsp coconut flour
1 Tbsp almond flour
½ tsp baking powder
Handful of blueberries or strawberries (optional)

Directions:

1. In a bowl, whisk the eggs with the milk, salt, xylitol, and melted butter (room temp.)
2. Add the coconut and almond flour to the mixture, along with the baking powder. Mix well.
3. Heat a non-stick pan over medium heat and scoop 3 Tbsp of the batter to make pancakes.
4. Flip the pancakes when bubbles start to form and cook until golden brown.
5. Serve with ½ cup of berries on the side.

(Calories 194.51 | Total Fats 13.4g | Net Carbs: 6.86g | Protein 31g)

Tomato Basil & Chili Scramble

(Total Time: 2 MIN| **Serve:** 10)

Ingredients:

4 egg whites
1 egg yolk
2 Tbsp almond milk
1 cup spinach
1 tomato, chopped
½ white onion, chopped
3 fresh basil leaves, chopped
¼ tsp of chili flakes
Salt and pepper to taste
Ghee

Directions:

1. In a bowl, whisk the egg yolk and whites with the milk. Stir well.
2. Heat the ghee in a pan over medium heat. Add the onions and sauté until fragrant.
3. Throw the tomato and chili into the pan with the spinach and cook until the spinach is almost wilted.
4. Pour the egg mixture over the spinach and cook until firm, or until the egg sets. Stir constantly.
5. Season with salt and pepper.
6. Serve warm

(Calories 203 | Total Fats 9g | Net Carbs: 2.86g | Protein 20g)

Mediterranean Egg Scramble

(Total Time: 10 MIN| Serve: 1)

Ingredients:

3 eggs
1 Tbsp pesto sauce
1 Tbsp olive oil
2 Tbsp sour cream
½ cup mashed avocado to serve

Directions:

1. Whisk the eggs in a bowl and season with salt and pepper.
2. Heat a non-stick pan over low heat. Drizzle with olive oil and pour the eggs into it. Constantly whisk the eggs while cooking.
3. Add the pesto mixture to the eggs and stir well.
4. Turn off the heat and mix in the sour cream. Combine well.
5. Serve with 1/2 cup mashed avocado.

(Calories 467.17 | Total Fats 41.12g | Net Carbs: 3.3g | Protein 20g)

Millet Gingerbread Mash

(Total Time: 10 MIN| **Serve:** 6)

Ingredients:

1 cup millet flour (or any kind of whole grain flour)
4 cups water
1/2 tsp ground ginger
1/4 tsp ground allspice
1/8 tsp ground nutmeg
1/4 tsp ground cardamom
1/4 tsp ground coriander
1 1/2 Tbsp ground cinnamon
1 tsp ground cloves
Sweetener of your choice (optional)

Directions:

1. In a medium saucepan bring water to boiling and cook the millet flour according to package directions. Add in all the spices together and stir.
2. Reduce heat and simmer, uncovered, for 5 minutes, stirring occasionally.
3. When cooked, add sweetener to taste and serve hot.

(Calories 58.18 | Total Fats 2.82g | Net Carbs: 0.2g | Protein 1.9g)

Scrambled Eggs with Bacon and Gouda Cheese

(Total Time: 15 MIN| **Serve:** 4)

Ingredients:

4 strips cooked bacon
4 eggs
2 1/2 Tbsp olive oil
1/4 cup softened cream cheese
1/4 cup shredded Gouda cheese
Garlic and onion powder
Black or white pepper

Directions:

1. In a frying pan, heat some olive oil and fry bacon slices until crisp.
2. In a small bowl beat the eggs with onion and garlic powder, cream cheese and shredded Gouda cheese. Season with salt and pepper to taste.
3. Pour egg mixture over bacon slices and cook for 3-4 minutes.
4. Serve and enjoy.

(Calories 380.72 | Total Fats 25.94g | Net Carbs: 0.95g | Protein 14.44g)

Nutty Cinnamon Granola

(Total Time: 25 MIN| **Serve:** 4)

Ingredients:

½ cup almonds

½ cup walnuts

½ cup hazelnuts, chopped

½ cup coconut flakes

½ cup mixed seeds (pumpkin seeds, flaxseeds, sunflower seeds, etc.)

2 tsp cinnamon, ground

3 Tbsp coconut oil, melted

Full cream yoghurt to serve

Directions:

1. Preheat oven at 350F.
2. Combine all the ingredients in a large bowl and stir well.
3. Transfer the mixture to a baking tray and place in the oven to cook for about 20 minutes. Shake every 5 minutes to make sure that the granola doesn't burn.
4. Let it cool and store in an airtight container.
5. Consume with a bowl of full-cream yogurt.

(Calories 210 | Total Fats 8g | Net Carbs: 30g | Protein 6g)

Baked Buckwheat Pancakes with Hazelnuts

(Total Time: 30 MIN| **Serve: 2**)

Ingredients:

1/2 cup buckwheat flour
3 eggs
1/2 cup coconut cream
1 vanilla bean (seeds only)
1 pinch of salt
3 Tbsp olive oil
Liquid sweetener of your choice
Hazelnuts

Directions:

1. Preheat oven to 400F degrees.
2. Grease an oval baking pan.
3. In a large bowl, add eggs, milk, flour, vanilla seeds, and salt. Mix the ingredients until the mixture becomes homogeneous (well blended).
4. Pour batter into prepared oval baking pan and spread evenly. Bake for 15-20 minutes.
5. Remove the pancake from the pan and serve with sweetener of your taste and hazelnuts.

(Calories 390.07 | Total Fats 22.66g | Net Carbs: 3.16g | Protein 14.4g)

Baked Parmesan-Almond Zucchini

(Total Time: 40 MIN| **Serve:** 6)

Ingredients:

2 zucchinis, thinly sliced to about 1-inch thick rounds
3 large eggs, beaten
1 cup almond flour
1 cup almonds, ground
1 cup grated Parmesan cheese
1 tsp dried oregano
Salt and pepper

Directions:

1. Preheat oven to 400 F degrees. Line a large baking sheet with parchment paper.
2. Wash, clean and slice zucchini. Salt from all sides and let dry on a paper towel. Set aside.
3. In abowl, combine ground almonds, Parmesan cheese, oregano and season with salt and pepper to taste and oregano; set aside.
4. In another shallow plate, add the almond flour.
5. In a third plate, beat eggs, with salt and pepper.
6. Start dredging zucchini rounds in flour, dip into eggs, then dredge in almond mixture, pressing to coat. Place zucchini slices on prepared baking sheet.
7. Bake for 20 to 30 minutes, or until the zucchini rounds are golden and crispy.
8. Serve hot.

(Calories 288.89 | Total Fats 17.49g | Net Carbs: 16.36g | Protein 12.12g)

Eggs with Motley Peppers and Zucchini

(Total Time: 25 MIN| **Serve:** 4)

Ingredients:

6 eggs
2 zucchini, diced
1 spring onion, chopped
1 green pepper, finely diced
1 yellow pepper, finely diced
1 red pepper, finely diced
3 Tbsp coconut oil (melted)
Salt and fresh ground black pepper to taste

Directions:

1. In a non-stick frying skillet, heat 2 Tbsp olive oil in a pan and sauté the onion for 5 minutes.
2. Add the peppers and fry for 2-3 minutes more.
3. Next, add the zucchini and sauté for another 3 minutes. Remove from heat and set aside.
4. In a medium bowl, beat the eggs with salt.
5. Mix the vegetables into the eggs.
6. Heat the remaining olive oil in the frying pan and pour in the egg and vegetable mixture.
7. Cook for 2-3 minutes constantly stirring.
8. Serve hot.

(Calories 165.31 | Total Fats 7.94g | Net Carbs: 6.55g | Protein 12.04g)

Kale, Peppers and Crumbled Feta Omelet

(Total Time: 3 HR 10 MIN| Serve: 4)

Ingredients:

8 eggs, well beaten
1 cup red peppers, diced
1/4 cup green onions (finely chopped)
1/2 cup crumbled Feta
3/4 cup kale, chopped
2 tsp olive oil
1/2 tsp Italian seasoning
Salt and freshly ground pepper, to taste
Sour cream cheese or cottage (optional)

Directions:

1. In a large frying pan heat oil on medium-high. Add chopped kale and cook about 3-4 minutes.
2. Wash and chop the red peppers. Slice the green onions and crumble the Feta. Grease the bottom of your Slow Cooker with olive oil. Add the chopped red pepper and sliced green onion to Slow Cooker with the kale.
3. In a small bowl, beat the eggs and pour over other ingredients in Slow Cooker. Stir well and add Italian seasonings. Adjust salt and pepper to taste.
4. Cook on LOW for 2 - 3 hours.

(Calories 279.34 | Total Fats 23.87g | Net Carbs: 1.16g | Protein 11.78g)

Mini Ham Omelettes Muffins

(Total Time: 25 MIN| **Serve:** 18)

Ingredients:

11 oz Ham Steak
10 green onions
12 Eggs
1/2 cup Heavy cream
9 slices mushrooms
9 slices Cheddar Cheese
Coconut oil for greasing
Salt, Pepper, Onion Powder, Garlic Powder to taste

Directions:

1. Preheat oven to 350F. Grease the muffin pan with coconut oil.
2. Dice the ham steak, slice the green onions and wash the mushrooms.
3. In a deep bowl, beat the eggs. Add in the heavy cream and spices along with ham cubes and sliced green onions.
4. Adjust salt, pepper, and spices to taste.
5. Fill each cavity of a muffin pan with the egg mixture.
6. Bake in the oven for 4-5 minutes.
7. Remove from the oven and add the mushrooms on the top
8. Cook for 8-9 more minutes or until the eggs are mostly set.
9. Add Cheddar cheese and cook for 1 more minute.
10. Serve hot.

(Calories 153.55| Total Fats 11.1g | Net Carbs: 0.59g | Protein 11.69g)

Nonpareil Bacon Waffles

(Total Time: 15 MIN| **Serve:** 2)

Ingredients:

4 slices bacon

2 eggs

3 cup almond flour

5 Tbsp melted butter or ghee

1 1/2 tsp baking powder

1 1/2 tsp sweetener of your choice

Directions:

1. Microwave the butter and set aside.
2. In a frying pan, cook the bacon until crisp.
3. Mix the dry ingredients first (almond flour, baking powder, and sweetener of your choice).
4. Add the two eggs and mix thoroughly. Add the melted butter and mix well.
5. Preheat the waffle maker.
6. When it is preheated, open and fill with batter and place 2 slices of bacon over the top.
7. Close and flip the waffle maker, when it beeps, flip it over and remove the waffle with a fork.
8. Serve hot.

(Calories 323.24 | Total Fats 24.97g | Net Carbs: 1.89g | Protein 8.35g)

Power Greens and Sausage Casserole

(Total Time: 1 HR 10 MIN| **Serve:** 10)

Ingredients:

12 eggs
1 1/4 lbs chicken or turkey sausage
1 cup kale leaves, chopped
1 cup arugula leaves, chopped
2 cups spinach, finely chopped
2 small zucchini - peeled
1 green onion, chopped
1/4 cup coconut milk
1/2 Tbsp coconut oil
1 tsp garlic powder
1 tsp sea salt
1 tsp pepper

Directions:

1. Heat oven to 365 F. Grease casserole dish with coconut oil.
2. In a frying pan, melt coconut oil over medium heat, Add in sausage and stir with a wooden spoon. Cook for two to three minutes.
3. In a big bowl, beat eggs.
4. Chop the green onion and peel the zucchini. Mix into eggs with seasoning, all greens, and coconut milk.
5. Pour egg mixture into casserole dish and stir in sausage. Adjust the salt and pepper to taste. Cook for 45 minutes.
6. Cover with foil and cook for 10-15 minutes more.
7. Serve hot.

(Calories 165.48 | Total Fats 7.98g | Net Carbs: 1.81g | Protein 12.19g)

Simple Bacon Pepper Pot

(Total Time: 25 MIN| Serve: 2)

Ingredients:

6 slices bacon
4 Eggs
1 small green pepper
Jalapeno pepper, sliced
1 green onion

Directions:

1. Slice the pepper, green onion and jalapeno into thin strips.
2. In a frying pan, cook the vegetables for about 2-3 minutes, until browned.
3. Chop the bacon in a food processor until it breaks into chunks.
4. Mix all the ingredients together.
5. Cook the hash until the bacon is becoming crisp.
6. Arrange on a plate and top with a fried egg!
7. Serve and enjoy.

(Calories 499.69 | Total Fats 29.87g | Net Carbs: 2.29g | Protein 23.33g)

Spinach-Chard Puree with Almonds

(Total Time: 35 MIN| **Serve:** 10)

Ingredients:

1 lb baby spinach leaves
1/2 lb Swiss chard, tough stems removed, tender stems and leaves torn into 2" pieces
1 cup cauliflower florets
1 leek
1/4 cup extra-virgin olive oil
3 cups water
4 Tbsp toasted almond slivers
1/4 cup tofu cheese, cubed
Salt and black ground pepper to taste

Directions:

1. Wash the leek and cut it into thick slices.
2. Heat the olive oil in a saucepan and cook the cauliflower and leek for about 2-3 minutes.
3. Add the chard and cleaned spinach leaves, water and a pinch of salt and pepper to taste. Bring to the boil and let it simmer for 15 minutes.
4. Remove from the heat and place the vegetables in a food processor. Blend into a very smooth soup.
5. Pour the mixture into bowls, place some tofu cubes on top and generously sprinkle with ground toasted almonds before serving

(Calories 47.47 | Total Fats 1.69g | Net Carbs: 0.94g | Protein 5.24g)

Buttermilk Seed Rusk's

(Total Time: 2 HR 40 MIN| **Serve:** 30)

Ingredients:

½ cup butter, melted
1 cup buttermilk
4 eggs
1 cup almond flour
1 cup ground flax
2 cups desiccated coconut
1 cup mixed seeds
2½ tsp baking powder
1 tsp salt
½ cup xylitol

Directions:

1. Preheat oven to 350 F.
2. In a bowl, combine thebuttermilk, butter, and eggs.
3. Slowly add the dry ingredients and stir well to make a batter.
4. Carefully transfer the mixture into a baking tray and cook in the oven for 45 minutes.
5. Allow to cool down before slicing it into 30 Rusk shapes.
6. Place on a wire rack upside down, and cook in the oven again for 90 minutes at 210F.

(Calories 119 | Total Fats 3g | Net Carbs: 17g | Protein 2g)

Ketogenic Mug Bread

(Total Time: 15 MIN| **Serve:** 3)

Ingredients:

1 Tbsp coconut flour
3 tbsp almond flour
1 tsp baking powder
1 whole egg
1 tsp melted butter
3 Tbsp water
A pinch of salt

Directions:

1. Add all the dry ingredients into a bowl, then add the egg and water and mix well. Make sure there are no lumps in your mixture.
2. Pour the melted butter into the cup you are going to use. You can also use the cup to melt the butter, to begin with, but make sure not to overheat the butter; 5 seconds in the microwave should be more than enough. Now swirl the butter around the cup making sure to coat the inside of the cup. Then pour the butter into the bread mixture and combine well.
3. Pour the mixture into your cup and microwave for 1.5 minutes. If you are planning on doubling the mixture, I would suggest using a bigger wider mug or the mixture will not cook all the way through. Don't microwave for more than 3 minutes or the mix will end up hard.
4. Once you have removed it from the mug, you can then slice it into rounds and place it in the toaster to crisp it up a little.

(Calories 238 | Total Fats 19g | Net Carbs: 2.6g | Protein 13g)

Lemon Cheesecake Breakfast Mousse

(Total Time: 10 MIN| **Serve**: 2)

Ingredients:

3 Tbsp cream cheese
1 Tbsp lemon juice
1.69 oz heavy cream (look for those with zero carbs)
3.38 oz Yoghurt
1 Tbsp xylitol
1/8 tsp salt
2 Tbsp whey protein powder
Berry coulis to serve

Directions:

1. Blend cream cheese and lemon juice in a bowl until smooth.
2. Add whey protein powder and mix well to avoid lumps.
3. Add heavy cream and blend until whipped. Gently fold in yogurt.
4. Taste and adjust sweetener if needed.
5. Serve with ¼ cup berry coulis.

(Calories 386 | Total Fats 19.8g | Net Carbs: 13.9g | Protein 34.4g)

Cacao and Raspberry Pudding

(Total **Time**: 40 MIN| **Serve**: 2)

Ingredients:

1 Tbsp cocoa powder
¼ cup raspberries
3 Tbsp chia seeds
1 cup almond milk
1 tsp agave nectar

Directions:

1. In a small bowl, combine the almond milk and cocoa powder. Stir well.
2. Add the chia seeds to the bowl and let it rest for 5 minutes.
3. Using a fork, fluff the chia and cocoa mixture and then place in the fridge to chill for at least 30 minutes.
4. Serve with raspberries and a drizzle of agave on top.

(Calories 402 | Total Fats 35.7g | Net Carbs: 21.2g | Protein 6.9g)

Mozzarella, Red Pepper & Bacon Frittata

(Total Time: 30 MIN| Serve: 6)

Ingredients:

9 eggs
1 Tbsp olive oil
2 Tbsp parsley, chopped
4 oz mozzarella cheese, cubed
1 red bell pepper, chopped
¼ cup heavy cream
7 bacon slices
4 caps large Bella mushrooms
½ cup basil, chopped
2 oz goat cheese, grated
¼ cup parmesan cheese, grated
Black pepper
Salt

Directions:

1. Set oven to 350 F.
2. Chop red pepper, bacon, basil, and mushroom. Slice mozzarella into cubes and put aside.
3. Heat olive oil in a skillet until it slightly smokes, then adds bacon and cook for 5 minutes until browned.
4. Add red pepper and cook for 2 minutes, until soft. While pepper cooks, add cream, parmesan cheese, eggs and black pepper to a bowl and whisk to combine.
5. Add mushrooms to pot with the bacon, stir and cook for 5 minutes until soaked in fat. Add basil, cook for 1 minute then add mozzarella.
6. Put in egg mixture and use a spoon to move ingredients around so that the egg gets on the bottom of the pan.
7. Top with goat cheese and place in oven for 8 minutes then broil for 6 minutes.
8. Use a knife to fry frittata edges from pan and place on a plate and slice.
9. Serve.

(Calories 408 | Total Fats 31.2g | Net Carbs: 2.4g | Protein 19.2g)

Rosemary, Sausage & Cheese Pies

(Total Time: 35 MIN| Serve: 2)

Ingredients:

¾ cup cheddar cheese, grated
¼ cup coconut oil
5 egg yolks
½ tsp rosemary
¼ tsp baking soda
1 ½ chicken sausage
¼ cup coconut flour
2 Tbsp coconut milk
2 tsp lemon juice
¼ tsp cayenne pepper
1/8 tsp kosher salt

Directions:

1. Set oven to 350 F.
2. Chop sausage, heat skillet and cook sausage.
3. While sausages cook combine all dry ingredients in a bowl.
4. In another bowl combine lemon juice, oil, and coconut milk. Add liquids to dry mixture and add ½ cup of cheese; fold to combine and put into 2 ramekins.
5. Add cooked sausages to the batter and use a spoon to submerge in the mixture.
6. Bake for 25 minutes, until golden on top. Top with leftover cheese and broil for 4 minutes.
7. Serve warm.

(Calories 711 | Total Fats 65.3g | Net Carbs: 5.8g | Protein 34.3g)

Pump-Cakes

(Total Time: 15 MIN| Serve: 2)

Ingredients:

¼ cup hazelnut flour
2 Tbsp egg white protein
1 tsp baking powder
1 Tbsp chai masala mix
½ cup pumpkin puree
3 free-range eggs
1 cup coconut cream
1 Tbsp stevia
Organic butter for cooking
Coconut cream for topping

Directions:

1. In a bowl, combine the hazelnut flour, egg white protein, baking protein, and chai masala mix, and Stevia. Stir well and set aside.
2. Using another mixing bowl, combine the pumpkin puree, eggs, and coconut cream. Blend the ingredients together until frothy, using a hand mixer.
3. Take the dry ingredients and then gradually whisk into the bowl with the pumpkin mixture.
4. The batter should be quite thick, but pourable. If the batter is too thick, add a few Tbsp of water.
5. Melt the butter in a non-stick pan over low heat.
6. Ladle the batter into the hot pan. Cover and cook for about 3 minutes on each side.
7. Serve the pump-cakes warm with a spoon of coconut cream on top.

(Calories 626 | Total Fats 58.3g | Net Carbs: 17.1g | Protein 16g)

Protein Loaded French bread

(Total Time: 15 MIN| **Serve:** 4)

Ingredients:

8 slices protein loaded bread
2 organic eggs
¼ cup coconut milk
1 tsp vanilla extract
1 tsp cinnamon powder
Coconut oil for frying

For the syrup:
½ cup organic butter
½ cup sugar replacement
½ cup almond milk, unsweetened

Directions:

1. Prepare the syrup by heating the butter in a saucepan. Wait for the butter to boil (be careful not to burn) and then pour the sugar replacement and almond milk into the saucepan. Whisk the ingredients together until smooth. Set aside to cool before transferring into a storage container.
2. In a bowl, whisk together the eggs, coconut milk, vanilla extract and cinnamon.
3. Dip the bread slices into the mixture and place into a hot non-stick skillet greased with coconut oil.
4. Toast the bread until brown on each side.
5. Repeat the same procedure until you've toasted all the bread slices.
6. Serve the French toast with a drizzle of the prepared syrup on top.

(Calories 265 | Total Fats 24.5g | Net Carbs: 1.5g | Protein 11.0g)

Fisherman's Breakfast

(Total Time: 15 MIN| Serve: 1)

Ingredients:

2 organic eggs
1 small jar sardines in olive oil
2 Tbsp artichoke hearts, cut into wedges
½ cup arugula
Salt and pepper to taste

Directions:

1. Set oven to 375 F.
2. Lay the sardines on an oven-proof dish. Break the eggs on top and then place a layer of the arugula leaves and artichokes.
3. Season with salt and pepper.
4. Place in the oven to cook for 10 minutes, or until the eggs are cooked through.
5. Serve hot.

(Calories 245 | Total Fats 15.2g | Net Carbs: 1.1g | Protein 25.1g)

Herbed Eggs

(Total Time: 20 MIN| Serve: 2)

Ingredients:

4 eggs
2 cloves of garlic, minced
1 tsp fresh thyme
½ fresh parsley, chopped
½ cup fresh cilantro, chopped
¼ tsp cayenne pepper, ground
¼ tsp cumin, ground
Salt to taste
2 tbsp organic butter

Directions:

1. Heat the butter in a non-stick pan over low heat.
2. Add the minced garlic into the hot pan and sauté for 3 minutes. Add the fresh thyme into the pan and cook for another half minute.
3. Throw in the chopped parsley and cilantro, stir, and cook for a further 3 minutes.
4. Carefully crack the eggs directly into the pan and cover. Add the seasonings.
5. Cook the eggs for 5-6 minutes, depending on your preferred doneness.
6. Serve with sausages or bacon on the side.

(Calories 299 | Total Fats 27.3g | Net Carbs: 3.2g | Protein 12g)

Smoked Salmon and Avocado Breakfast

(Total Time: 10 MIN| Serve: 2)

Ingredients:

1 ripe avocado, peel removed and cut into cubes
¼ cup smoked salmon
2 Tbsp softened goat cheese
2 Tbsp ghee
2 Tbsp lemon juice
Salt to taste

Directions:

1. Cut the avocado into cubes and place in serving bowl.
2. Add the smoked salmon and carefully fold together with a spoon.
3. Add the rest of the ingredients and combine.
4. Season with salt before serving.

(Calories 366 | Total Fats 35.1g | Net Carbs: 9.1g | Protein 7.6g)

Creamy Greens Breakfast Pie

(Total Time: 45 MIN| **Serve:** 4)

Ingredients:

1 lb. sausage meat
8 cups baby spinach
3 organic eggs
1 cup mozzarella, shredded
2 cups ricotta cheese
¼ cup parmesan cheese, shredded
1 Tbsp organic butter
1 clove of garlic, minced
1 small onion, chopped
1/8 tsp nutmeg, ground
Salt and pepper

Directions:

1. Set the oven at 350 F.
2. Heat the butter in a pan over medium heat. Sauté the onion and garlic for 3-4 minutes.
3. Add the baby spinach into the pan and cook for another 5 minutes, or until the leaves wilt.
4. Season with nutmeg, salt, and pepper. Stir and turn off the heat. Set aside.
5. Beat the eggs in a large bowl and whisk in all the cheeses. Mix well.
6. Add the cooked greens in the bowl with the eggs and combine.
7. Meanwhile, place the sausage meat into a baking dish, press and mold it into a pie crust.
8. Pour the egg and spinach mixture into the pie crust and place in the oven to cook for 35 minutes, or until the eggs are firm. Remember to place a baking sheet below the baking dish, so you do not end up with a messy oven.

(Calories 584 | Total Fats 42.7g | Net Carbs: 9.4g | Protein 40.2g)

Sausage Biscuits

(Total Time: 35 MIN| Serve: 4)

Ingredients:

½ cup softened cream cheese

1 organic egg

2 cloves of garlic, minced

1 Tbsp chives, chopped

Salt to taste

½ tsp Italian seasoning

1 cup sharp cheddar cheese, shredded

¼ cup heavy cream

1½ cups almond flour

¼ cup water

½ lb. cooked ground sausage

Directions:

1. Set the oven at 350 F.
2. In a bowl, whip the softened cream cheese and eggs using a hand mixer. Add the minced garlic, chives, salt, and Italian seasoning into the bowl and carefully mix together.
3. Also add in the cheddar, heavy cream, almond flour and water into the mixture. Combine well with a metal spoon.
4. Take the cooked ground sausage and gradually add it to the cream cheese mixture, stirring to blend well.
5. Prepare a muffin pan by greasing it with oil or butter and then fill the muffin cups (about 8) with the prepared mixture.
6. Place in the oven to bake for 25 minutes.
7. Allow the biscuits to cool before removing from the pan and serving.

(Calories 437| Total Fats 37.7g | Net Carbs: 2.3g | Protein 21.9g)

Olives and Avocado Frittata

(Total Time: 15 MIN| **Serve:** 2)

Ingredients:

4 organic eggs
1 ripe avocado, cut into thick slices
10 olives, pitted
½ cup brie cheese, sliced thin
1 tsp Italian seasoning
2 Tbsp ghee
2 Tbsp olive oil
Salt to taste

Directions:

1. In a large mixing bowl, whisk together the eggs, olives, Italian seasoning, and salt. Whisk until frothy. Set aside.
2. In a non-stick skillet, add the ghee and heat over mediumheat before adding the avocado slices and frying until golden brown. Set aside.
3. Using the same pan, increase the heat to high and pour in the egg mixture.
4. Add the brie cheese into the pan, cover and cook for 3 minutes.
5. Flip the frittata and cook for another 2-3 minutes.
6. Serve the frittata with the fried avocados on top.

(Calories 690 | Total Fats 65.7g | Net Carbs: 9.7g | Protein 20.5g)

Cheesy Cauliflower Waffle

(Total Time: 15 MIN| **Serve:** 2)

Ingredients:

¾ cup cauliflower florets
2 organic eggs
¼ cup cheddar
¼ cup mozzarella
1 Tbsp chives
¼ tsp onion powder
¼ tsp garlic powder
Salt and pepper to taste

Directions:

1. Place the cauliflower, cheddar, and mozzarella in a food processor and pulse until all the ingredients are chopped and mixed.
2. Add the eggs and the rest of the ingredients into the food processor and blend. Make sure that the ingredients are well-combined.
3. Heat your waffle maker and pour the mixture in it to cook, based on the time which the waffle maker instructions recommend.
4. Serve the waffles warm with cream cheese and bacon on the side.

(Calories 140 | Total Fats 7.9g | Net Carbs: 3.7g | Protein 13.9g)

Eggs n' Steak Breakfast

(Total Time: 15 MIN| Serve: 5)

Ingredients:

2 lbs. beef chuck shoulder
7 organic eggs
1 small onion, chopped
1 bell pepper, chopped
¼ cup cheddar cheese, shredded
½ cup heavy cream
½ tsp garlic powder
Salt and pepper to taste
½ tbsp butter

Directions:

1. Add butter in a pan and melt over medium heat.
2. Add the onion and bell peppers and cook for 4-5 minutes. Set aside.
3. Place the same pan back on the stove and increase the heat to high. Add the steaks to the pan and cook for 6 minutes on each side. Set the steaks aside to rest.
4. In a large bowl, mix together the eggs, heavy cream, garlic powder, salt, and pepper.
5. Cook the egg mixture in a hot non-stick pan and stir occasionally.
6. Transfer the cooked eggs to a serving plate and serve with the sliced steaks on the side.

(Calories 506 | Total Fats 51g | Net Carbs: 4g | Protein 45g)

Keto Breakfast Biscuit

(Total Time: 15 MIN| **Serve:** 2)

Ingredients:

2 large eggs, (separate the white and yolk of one egg)
¼ cup softened cream cheese
2 Tbsp parmesan cheese, grated
½ tsp psyllium husks
½ tsp organic apple cider vinegar
A pinch of baking powder
A pinch of garlic powder
Salt and pepper to taste
1 tsp olive oil, plus a ½ tsp. for cooking
1 slice of American cheese cut in half

Directions:

1. In a bowl, whisk together the egg white from one egg, cream cheese, parmesan, psyllium husks, apple cider, baking powder, and garlic powder. Combine well.
2. Brush 2 ramekins with the olive oil and pour the prepared batter. Place in the microwave to cook for 35 seconds on high.
3. Heat the leftover oil in a non-stick pan and add the remaining egg plus the yolk from the other egg, and fry until over medium.
4. Place the cheese slices and fried eggs on top of the cooked biscuits and serve immediately.

(Calories 68 | Total Fats 9.9g | Net Carbs: 4.3g | Protein 8.3g)

Bacon Hash and Eggs

(Total Time: 15 MIN| Serve: 2)

Ingredients:

4 organic eggs
6 bacon strips, cooked
1 onion, chopped
1 green bell pepper, chopped
1 Tbsp jalapenos, diced
1 Tbsp ghee

Directions:

1. Heat the ghee in a cast iron skillet over medium heat. Add the chopped onions, bell pepper, and jalapenos, and sauté until the onions become translucent. Set aside.
2. Chop the cooked the bacon and mix into the cooked vegetables.
3. Place egg rings into a pan with oil and then scoop the veggie and bacon mixture into the rings.
4. Cook until the hash is almost crispy. Set aside.
5. Fry the eggs in a pan and serve on top of the bacon hash.

(Calories 366 | Total Fats 24g | Net Carbs: 11g | Protein 23g)

Bacon Waffles

(Total Time: 15 MIN| **Serve:** 2)

Ingredients:

4 bacon strips, cooked crispy chopped
2 organic eggs
5 Tbsp organic butter, melted
¾ cup almond flour
1 ½ tsp stevia
1 ½ tsp baking powder
Whipped cream (as topping)

Directions:

1. In a bowl, combine the flour, stevia, and baking powder together.
2. Crack the eggs into the bowl and combine well.
3. Pour in the melted butter and mix again. Set aside.
4. Heat your waffle maker and set it on medium.
5. Grease the waffle maker before pouring in the batter.
6. Sprinkle the bacon crisps on top and then cook according to equipment instructions.
7. Serve with whipped cream on top.

(Calories 648 | Total Fats 61g | Net Carbs: 10g | Protein 21g)

Ham and Cheese Omelet

(Total Time: 20 MIN| **Serve:** 4)

Ingredients:

5.29 oz ham, diced
6 organic eggs
½ cup heavy cream
¼ tsp pepper
¼ tsp salt
¼ tsp garlic powder
½ cup diced tomatoes
6 green onions, chopped
4 slices cheddar cheese

Directions:

1. Set the oven 350 F.
2. In a large bowl, combine the eggs, heavy cream, and season with salt, pepper, and garlic powder. Add the diced ham and tomatoes before stirring well.
3. Pour egg mixture into a greased muffin tin.
4. Place in the oven to cook for 5 minutes.
5. Remove the tin from the oven and then add the green onions on top.
6. Place in the oven to cook for another 8 minutes.
7. Remove again from the oven and place the cheese slices on top, and bake again for another minute.
8. Serve warm.

(Calories 257 | Total Fats 18g | Net Carbs: 4g | Protein 17g)

Egg-Stuffed Meat Balls

(Total Time: 60 MIN| Serve: 4)

Ingredients:

4 organic eggs, cooked hard boiled
12oz. ground pork sausage
8 bacon slices

Directions:

1. Divide the ground sausage into four and form into patties.
2. Place the hardboiled egg in the middle of the patties (one each), and cover the egg with the ground pork.
3. Place in the fridge to chill for at least 30 minutes.
4. Set oven to 450 F.
5. Take 2 bacon slices and wrap around the meatballs and secure with toothpicks.
6. Place on a baking sheet and bake in the oven to cook for 20 minutes or until the bacon is crisp.
7. Serve immediately.

(Calories 351 | Total Fats 28.5g | Net Carbs: 0.3g | Protein 22.1g)

Cheeseburger Quiche

(Total Time: 40 MIN| **Serve:** 8)

Ingredients:

4 organic eggs
¼ lb. bacon
½ lb. ground beef
1 onion, chopped
½ cup mayonnaise
½ cup heavy cream
2 cups sharp cheddar cheese, shredded
Salt and pepper to taste

Directions:

1. Set the oven at 350 F.
2. Cook the bacon to a crisp and set aside.
3. Using the same pan, sauté the onions, add ground beef and cook until done.
4. Meanwhile, combine the eggs, mayonnaise, and heavy cream in a bowl. Season with salt and pepper; mix well.
5. Chop the cooked bacon and add to the bowl.
6. Also, add the cooked ground beef and mix well.
7. Add half of the cheese to the mixture and stir again.
8. Pour the meat and egg mixture into a baking dish into a greased baking dish, top with the rest of the cheese, and place in the oven to bake for 30 minutes, or until the eggs are cooked through.
9. Allow to cool for at least 10 minutes before serving.

(Calories 532 | Total Fats 44g | Net Carbs: 5g | Protein 27g)

Vegan-Friendly Scramble

(Total Time: 30 MIN| Serve: 2)

Ingredients:

2 tbsp olive oil
2 cloves of garlic, chopped
1 onion, chopped
½ lb. firm tofu, remove excess liquid and chop into cubes
¼ tsp cinnamon, ground
1 Tbsp chili powder
Salt and pepper to taste
1 tsp organic apple cider vinegar
2 Tbsp fresh cilantro, chopped

Directions:

1. Heat the olive oil in a non-stick pan and sauté the onions and garlic for 3-5 minutes.
2. Add the tofu into the pan and crumble.
3. Stir the tofu with the onion and garlic and season with cinnamon, chili powder, salt, and pepper.
4. Cook for 15-20 minutes, or until the tofu is done.
5. Turn off the heat and immediately add the apple cider.
6. Place the tofu scramble into serving bowls and garnish with chopped cilantro.

(Calories 239 | Total Fats 19.5g | Net Carbs: 10.4g | Protein 10.6g)

Bacon and Peanut Butter Muffin Cups

(Total Time: 25 MIN| Serve: 4)

Ingredients:

2 tbsp all-natural peanut butter
2 bacon strips, cooked and chopped
1 cup almond flour
1 tsp baking powder
1 organic egg
2 Tbsp heavy cream
1 tsp vanilla extract

Directions:

1. Set oven to 350 F.
2. In a bowl, mix together the almond flour and baking powder.
3. Beat the egg lightly and add to the dry ingredients.
4. Also add the heavy cream, vanilla extract, chopped bacon, and all-natural peanut butter. Stir well.
5. Pour the batter into greased muffin tins and place in the oven to bake for 15 minutes, or until the toothpick comes out clean after being inserted into the muffins.
6. Serve warm.

(Calories 270 | Total Fats 23g | Net Carbs: 8g | Protein 10g)

Sweet, Salty, and Savory Crepe

(Total Time: 20 MIN| Serve: 2)

Ingredients:

3 organic eggs
½ cup softened cream cheese
½ Tbsp stevia
½ tsp cinnamon powder
4 slices ham
4 slices deli turkey
1 cup Swiss cheese, grated
2 Tbsp organic butter (divided into 2)

Directions:

1. Place the first four ingredients in a food processor and pulse until you achieve a nice batter. Set aside and let it rest for 5 minutes.
2. Melt the butter in a non-stick pan over the medium-high heat and scoop a heaped Tbsp of the batter into the pan. Move the pan from side to side in a circular motion to create a crepe. Cook each side for 2 minutes.
3. Assemble the crepe by topping with 1 slice of ham, 1 slice of deli turkey, and sprinkle with the Swiss cheese.
4. Place another crepe on top and do the same procedure.
5. Using the same pan, melt the remaining butter and then place the stacked crepe into it. Cover and allow to cook for 2 minutes before flipping the crepe. You're done the cooking when the cheese is starting to melt.
6. Serve warm.

(Calories 825 | Total Fats 67g | Net Carbs: 6g | Protein 57g)

Eggs Benedict

(Total Time: 20 MIN| **Serve:** 2)

Ingredients:

8 organic eggs
2 egg yolks
8 strips of bacon, cooked
2 cups baby spinach
1 juice of lemon
1 Tbsp water
1 cup melted butter
¼ tsp salt
½ tsp pepper
½ tsp Worcestershire sauce

Directions:

1. Prepare a double boiler on medium-low heat. In the top pot, combine the yolks, lemon juice, Worcestershire sauce, pepper and a tbsp of water. Whisk well with a hand whisk and set the thickened sauce aside.
2. Gradually add the melted butter in the pot, whisking all the time.
3. Meanwhile, crack an egg into a mug and zap in the microwave for a minute. Do the same thing with the rest of the 7 eggs.
4. Place the baby spinach on a serving plate and top with the chopped Canadian bacon, the microwaved eggs, and drizzle with the Hollandaise sauce.

(Calories 252 | Total Fats 53.6g | Net Carbs: 6.4g | Protein 15g)

Almond Bread

(Total Time: 25 MIN| **S**erve: 8)

Ingredients:

2 eggs
1 cup almond butter, unsalted
3/4 cup almond flour
1 Tbsp cinnamon
1 tsp pure vanilla extract
1/4 tsp baking soda
2 Tbsp liquid stevia
1/2 tsp sea salt

Directions:

1. Preheat oven to 340 F degrees.
2. In a deep bowl whisk eggs, almond butter, honey, stevia, and vanilla. Add in almond flour, salt, cinnamon, and baking soda. Stir until all ingredients are well combined.
3. Pour dough into a greased baking pan. Bake for 12-15 minutes.
4. Once ready, let cool on a wire rack. Slice and serve.

(Calories 208.6 | Total Fats 16.7g | Net Carbs: 7.64g | Protein 15g)

Chapter 5: Poultry

Chicken Pie

(Total Time: 30 MIN| Serve: 5)

Ingredients:

½ lb. boneless chicken thighs cut into small pieces
3.5 oz bacon, chopped
1 carrot, chopped
¼ cup parsley, chopped
1 cup heavy cream
2 onion leeks, chopped
1 cup white wine
1 Tbsp olive oil
Salt and pepper to taste

__For the crust__
1 cup almond meal
2 Tbsp water
1 Tbsp stevia
1½ Tbsp butter
½ tsp salt

Directions:

1. Prepare the crust first by combining all its ingredients to make a crumbly textured dough. Set aside.
2. Heat the olive oil in a pan on medium-high. Throw in the chopped leeks and stir until a bit soft. Transfer to a plate.
3. Throw in the chicken meat and bacon and cook until brown and then add the leeks.
4. Add the carrots and pour the white wine and then reduce the heat to medium.
5. Add the parsley and the heavy cream and stir well. Transfer into a baking dish.
6. Cover with the prepared crumb crust and place in the oven to cook until the crust turns golden brown and crispy.
7. Allow resting for 20 minutes before serving.

(Calories 396| Total Fats 33g | Net Carbs: 6.5g | Protein 12.1g)

Classic Chicken Parmigiana

(Total Time: 50 MIN| **Serve**: 2)

Ingredients:

2 boneless chicken thighs
8 strips of bacon, chopped
½ cup parmesan cheese, grated
½ cup mozzarella cheese, shredded
1 organic egg
1 can diced tomato

Directions:

1. Set the oven at 450 F.
2. Tenderize the chicken with a meat mallet and set aside.
3. Place the parmesan cheese on a plate.
4. Crack the egg into a bowl and whisk. Dip the chicken into it.
5. Then coat the chicken with the parmesan.
6. Grease the baking sheet with butter, place the chicken thighs onto it and bake in the oven for 30-40 minutes.
7. While waiting for the chicken to bake, cook the bacon.
8. Pour the tomatoes in with the bacon and stir. Reduce the heat to low and allow simmering and reducing.
9. Remove the chicken from the oven when done and ladle over the reduced tomato sauce.
10. Sprinkle with the mozzarella on top and place back in the oven to melt the cheese.
11. Serve hot.

(Calories 826 | Total Fats 50.3g | Net Carbs: 6.2g | Protein 83.2g)

Turkey Leg Roast

(Total Time: 1 HR 20 MIN| **Serve:** 4)

Ingredients:

2 turkey legs
2 Tbsp ghee

For the rub:
¼ tsp cayenne
½ tsp thyme, dried
½ tsp ancho chili powder
½ tsp garlic powder
½ tsp onion powder
1 tsp liquid smoke
1 tsp Worcestershire
Salt and pepper to taste

Directions:

1. Set the oven at 350 F.
2. Combine all the ingredients for the rub in a bowl. Whisk well.
3. Dry the turkey legs with a clean towel and generously rub with the spice mixture.
4. Heat the ghee on medium-high in a cast iron skillet and then sear the turkey legs for 2 minutes on each side.
5. Place the turkey in the oven to bake for one hour.

(Calories 382 | Total Fats 22.5g | Net Carbs: 0.8g | Protein 44g)

Slow-Cooked Greek Chicken

(Total Time: 7 HR 10 MIN| **S**erve: 4)

Ingredients:

4 boneless chicken thighs
3 cloves of garlic, minced
3 Tbsp lemon juice
1 ½ cups hot water
2 cubes chicken bouillon
3 Tbsp Greek Rub

Directions:

1. Coat the slow cooker with cooking spray
2. Season the chicken with the Greek rub followed by the minced garlic.
3. Transfer the chicken to the slow cooker and sprinkle with lemon juice on top.
4. Crumble the chicken cubes and put in the slow cooker. Pour the water in and stir.
5. Cover and cook on low for 6-7 hours.
6. Uncover and serve with vegetables or salad.

(Calories 140 | Total Fats 5.7g | Net Carbs: 2.2g | Protein 18.6g)

Roasted Bacon-Wrapped Chicken

(Total Time: 1 HR 25 MIN| **S**erve: 6)

Ingredients:

1 whole dressed chicken
10 strips of bacon
3 sprigs fresh thyme
2 lime wedges
Salt and pepper to taste

Directions:

1. Set the oven at 500 F.
2. Thoroughly rinse the chicken and stuff it with the lime wedges and thyme sprigs.
3. Season the chicken with salt and pepper and then wrap the chicken with the bacon.
4. Season again with salt and pepper and then place on a roasting tray on top of a baking sheet (make sure to catch the juices) and place in the oven to roast for 15 minutes.
5. Lower the temperature to 350 F and then roast for another 45 minutes.
6. Remove the chicken from the oven, cover with foil and set aside for 15 minutes.
7. Take the juices from the tray and place in a saucepan. Bring to a boil over high heat and use an immersion blender to mix all the "good stuff" from the juice.
8. Serve the chicken with the sauce on the side.

(Calories 375 | Total Fats 29.8g | Net Carbs: 2.4g | Protein 24.5g)

Crispy Curried Chicken

(Total Time: 60 MIN| **Serve: 4**)

Ingredients:

4 chicken thighs
¼ cup olive oil
1 tsp curry powder
¼ tsp ginger
½ tsp cumin, ground
½ tsp smoked paprika
½ tsp garlic powder
¼ tsp cayenne
¼ tsp allspice
¼ Tbsp chili powder
Pinch of coriander, ground
Pinch of cinnamon
Pinch of cardamom
½ tsp salt

Directions:

1. Set the oven at 425 F.
2. Combine all the spices together.
3. Line a baking sheet with foil and lay the chicken on it.
4. Drizzle the chicken with olive oil, and rub.
5. Sprinkle the spice mixture on top and then rub again, make sure to coat the chicken with the spices.
6. Place in the oven to bake for 50 minutes.
7. Allow to rest for 5 minutes before serving.

(Calories 277 | Total Fats 19.9g | Net Carbs: 0.6g | Protein 42.3g)

The Perfect Baked Chicken Wings

(Total Time: 40 MIN| **Serve:** 2)

Ingredients:

2.5 lbs chicken wings
½ tsp baking soda
1 tsp baking powder
Salt to taste
4 tbsp butter, melted

Directions:

1. Add all the ingredients (except butter) in a Ziploc bag and shake, making sure that the wings are coated with the mixture.
2. Place in the fridge overnight.
3. When you're ready to cook, set the oven at 450 F.
4. Place the wings on a baking sheet and cook in the oven for 20 minutes.
5. Flip the wings and bake for another 15 minutes.
6. Melt the butter and drizzle over the wings.

(Calories 500 | Total Fats 0.0g | Net Carbs: 38.8g | Protein 44g)

Chicken in Kung Pao Sauce

(Total Time: 25 MIN| **Serve: 2**)

Ingredients:

2 boneless chicken thighs cut into smaller pieces
½ green pepper, chopped
2 spring onions, sliced thin
¼ cup peanuts, chopped
1 tsp ginger, grated
½ Tbsp red chili flakes
Salt and pepper to taste

For the sauce:
2 tsp rice wine vinegar
1 Tbsp keto Ketchup
2 Tbsp chili garlic paste
1 Tbsp low-sodium soy sauce
2 tsp sesame oil
2 tsp liquid stevia
½ tsp maple syrup

Directions:

1. Season the chicken with salt, pepper, and grated ginger.
2. Place a cast iron skillet over the medium-high fire and add the chicken when the pan is hot. Cook for 10 minutes.
3. Whisk all the ingredients for the sauce in a bowl while waiting for the chicken to cook.
4. Add the green pepper, spring onions, and peanuts to the pan with the chicken, and cook for another 4-5 minutes
5. Add the sauce to the pan stir and bring to the boil before serving ladled generously over the chicken.

(Calories 362 | Total Fats 27.4g | Net Carbs: 3.2g | Protein 22.3g)

Chicken BBQ Pizza

(Total Time: 20 MIN| **Serve:** 4)

Ingredients:

1 cup roasted chicken, shredded
4 Tbsp BBQ sauce
½ cup cheddar cheese
1 Tbsp mayonnaise
4 Tbsp all-natural tomato sauce

For the keto pizza crust
6 Tbsp parmesan cheese, grated
6 organic eggs
3 Tbsp psyllium husk powder
2 Tsp Italian seasoning
Salt and pepper to taste

Directions:

1. Set oven to 425 F.
2. Place all the ingredients for the crust in a food processor and pulse until you achieve a thick dough.
3. Shape the pizza dough and place in the oven to cook for 10 minutes.
4. Top the cooked crust with the tomato sauce followed by the chicken, cheese, and a drizzle of the BBQ sauce and mayonnaise on top.
5. Place in the oven for 10 more minutes, or untilt he cheese is melted and bubbling.
6. Cut into wedges and serve.

(Calories 357 | Total Fats 24.5g | Net Carbs: 2.9g | Protein 24.5g)

Slow Cooked Chicken Masala

(Total Time: 3 HR 10 MIN| Serve: 2)

Ingredients:

1 ½ lb. boneless chicken thighs, sliced into small pieces
2 cloves of garlic
1 tsp ginger, grated
1 tsp onion powder
3 Tbsp masala
1 tsp paprika
2 tsp salt
½ cup coconut milk (divided into 2)
2 Tbsp tomato paste
½ cup diced tomatoes
2 Tbsp olive oil
½ cup heavy cream
1 tsp stevia
Fresh cilantro for garnish

Directions:

1. Place the chicken in the slow cooker first. Add the grated ginger, garlic, and the rest of the spices. Stir.
2. Add the tomato paste and diced tomatoes next and stir again.
3. Pour the ½ of the coconut milk and mix, cover and then cook on high for 3 hours.
4. When the cooking is done, uncover and add the remaining coconut milk, heavy cream, stevia, and mix again.
5. Serve hot.

(Calories 493 | Total Fats 41.2g | Net Carbs: 5.8g | Protein 26g)

Baked Buttered Chicken

(Total Time: 1 HR 10 MIN| Serve: 2)

Ingredients:

4 chicken thighs

¼ cup softened organic butter

1 tsp rosemary, dried

1 tsp basil, dried

½ tsp salt

½ tsp pepper

Directions:

1. Set oven to 350 F.
2. Whisk all the ingredients (except the chicken) in a bowl.
3. Place the chicken thighs on a baking sheet lined with foil and generously brush it with the butter mixture.
4. Place the chicken in the oven to bake for an hour.
5. Serve warm.

(Calories 735 | Total Fats 33.7g | Net Carbs: 0.8g | Protein 101.8g)

Chicken, Bacon & Cream Cheese Pot Pie

(Total Time: 25 MIN| Serve: 8)

Ingredients:

For filling:

5 bacon slices
1 tsp garlic powder
8 oz cream cheese
6 cups spinach
Salt
6 chicken thighs, boneless and skinless
1 tsp onion powder
¾ tsp celery seed
4 oz cheddar cheese
¼ cup chicken broth

For crust:

3 Tbsp psyllium husk powder
1 egg
¼ cup cheddar cheese
¼ tsp garlic powder
Salt
1/3 cup almond flour
3 Tbsp butter
¼ cup cream cheese
½ tsp paprika
¼ tsp onion powder
Black pepper

Directions:

1. Cube chicken and season with black pepper and salt.
2. Set oven to 375 F.
3. Use spices to season chicken and place into an oven proof skillet and cook on medium-high, until golden on the outside. Add bacon to pan and cook until golden.

4. Add broth to the pan, along with cheeses and stir to combine. Put spinach in the pan and cook until wilted.
5. Combine dry ingredients for crust in a bowl and set aside.
6. Put cheddar and cream cheese into a microwave safe dish and warm slightly before addingegg and combine well. Add mixture to dry ingredients and mix together to form a dough for the crust.
7. Stir ingredients in pot and top with crust and use fork to pierce crust all over.
8. Bake for 15 minutes, take from oven and cool.
9. Serve.

(Calories 434 | Total Fats 35.6g | Net Carbs: 3.4g | Protein 20.4g)

Chicken Hash

(Total **Time:** 30 MIN| **Serve:** 2)

Ingredients:

1 Tbsp olive oil
1/4 onion finely diced
1 cups broccoli
1 cup chicken stock
1.7 oz chicken breast cooked and finely diced
½ tsp salt
¼ tsp black pepper
¼ cup pumpkin

Directions:

1. Add all ingredients to chicken stock, cover and cook approximately 20 minutes.
2. Spoon onto serving plates and serve.

(Calories 125 | Total Fats 8g | Net Carbs: 7g | Protein 7g)

Chicken Parmesan

(Total Time: 25 MIN| **S**erve: 4)

Ingredients:

For Chicken:
3 chicken breasts
1 cup mozzarella cheese
Salt
Black pepper

For coating:
¼ cup flaxseed meal
1 tsp oregano
½ tsp black pepper
½ tsp garlic powder
1 Egg
2.5 oz pork rinds
½ cup parmesan cheese
½ tsp salt
¼ tsp red pepper flakes
2 tsp paprika
1 ½ tsp chicken broth

For Sauce:
1 cup tomato sauce, low carb
2 garlic cloves
Salt
½ cup olive oil
½ tsp oregano
Black pepper

Directions:

1. Add flax meal, spices, pork rinds and parmesan cheese in a processor and grind until combined.

2. Pound chicken breast to flatten and whisk egg together with broth in a container.
3. Add all ingredients for the sauce to a pan, stir and put over a low flame to cook.
4. Dip chicken in egg mixture and then coat with dry mixture.
5. Heat oil in a pan and fry chicken, then transfer to a casserole dish.
6. Top with sauce and mozzarella and bake for 10 minutes.
7. Serve.

(Calories 646 | Total Fats 46.8g | Net Carbs: 4g | Protein 49.3g)

Chicken Stir-Fry

(Total Time: 20 MIN| **Serve**: 4)

Ingredients:

4 chicken breasts (butterflied), marinated in egg white overnight

2 cups red pepper

2 cups mange tout

2 cups grated carrot

2 cups broccoli

2 cups almonds

2 cloves of garlic

½ tsp ginger

2 Tbsp soya sauce

¾ cup chicken stock

2 Tbsp coconut oil

Directions:

1. Heat coconut oil in a pan over medium heat. Sauté the garlic and ginger until fragrant.
2. Cook the chicken breast in the oil and then add the vegetables. Toss and cook until almost done.
3. Add 2 Tbsp. soya sauce and 125ml chicken stock. Allow to simmer uncovered until the broth evaporates.

(Calories 186 | Total Fats 11g | Net Carbs: 4g | Protein 17g)

Nacho Chicken Casserole

(Total Time: 45 MIN| Serve: 4)

Ingredients:

1 ½ tsp chili seasoning
4 oz cream cheese
1 cup tomatoes and green chilies
¼ cup sour cream
1 jalapeno pepper
1 ¾ lbs chicken thigh, skinless and boneless
2 Tbsp olive oil
4 oz cheddar cheese
3 tbsp parmesan cheese
1 pack cauliflower, frozen
Salt
Black pepper

Directions:

1. Set oven to 375 F.
2. Season chicken with pepper and salt, heat oil in a skillet and cook chicken for 5-7 minutes until golden all over.
3. Add sour cream, ¾ cheddar cheese, and cream cheese to chicken. Stir until combined and cheeses are melted. Add tomatoes and combine before transferring to a casserole dish.
4. Place cauliflower in a microwave safe dish and cook thoroughly. Add leftover cheese and use a masher or immersion blender to combine into a smooth puree. Add pepper and salt to taste.
5. Spread mixture on top of chicken mixture and top with jalapenos.
6. Bake for 20 minutes.
7. Serve warm.

(Calories 426 | Total Fats 32.2g | Net Carbs: 4.3g | Protein 30.8g)

Kung Pao Chicken

(Total Time: 45 MIN| Serve: 3)

Ingredients:

For sauce:
2 tsp rice wine vinegar
1 Tbsp ketchup, low sugar
½ tsp maple extract
1 Tbsp soy sauce
2 Tbsp garlic chili paste
2 tsp sesame oil
10 drops liquid stevia

For chicken:
1 tsp ground ginger
¼ cup peanuts
2 spring onions
2 chicken thighs
Salt
Black pepper
½ green pepper, sliced
4 bird's eye peppers, seeds removed

Directions:

1. Chop chicken thighs and heat oil in a skillet. Add chicken to the pot and cook for 10 minutes.
2. Add remaining ingredients for chicken and cook for 5 minutes, before adding peanuts and vegetables and cooking for an additional 5 minutes.
3. Combine sauce ingredients and add to chicken. Cook for 10 minutes, or until sauce reduces.
4. Spoon in bowls and serve.

(Calories 362 | Total Fats 27.4g | Net Carbs: 3.2g | Protein 22.3g)

Chipotle Blackberry Wings

(Total Time: 1 HR 30 MIN| **Serve:** 5)

Ingredients:

For Jam:
8 oz Blackberries
¼ cup erythritol
¼ cup MCT oil
1 ½ chipotle in adobo
8 drops liquid stevia
¼ tsp guar gum

For Chicken:
20 Chicken wings
½ cup Water
½ cup Blackberry jam
Salt
Pepper

Directions:

1. Prepare sauce (may be made from the day before). Place berries in a saucepan and heat until softened.
2. Add erythritol, stevia, and chipotle; mash together to combine and add oil. Boil for 8 minutes, then add gum and combine. Strain and put aside to cool and refrigerate.
3. Separate wings into wings and drumettes, saving tips for other use.
4. Add blackberry jam to a bowl with water and mix, remove 1/3 of sauce and set aside for later basting. Add wings to remaining sauce in bowl. Add pepper and salt to taste; refrigerate for 30 minutes or more.
5. Set oven to 400F.
6. Bake for 15 minutes, turn over, coat with leftover sauce and bake for an additional 30 minutes.
7. Serve on individual plates with a finger bowl nearby to wash your sticky fingers.

(Calories 503 | Total Fats 39.1g | Net Carbs: 1.8g | Protein 34.5g)

Jalapeno Chicken Casserole

(Total Time: 1 HR 15 MIN| **Serve:** 6)

Ingredients:

6 bacon slices
12 oz cream cheese
4 oz cheddar cheese, shredded
¼ cup hot sauce
6 chicken thighs
3 jalapenos, seeds removed
¼ cup mayonnaise
2 oz mozzarella cheese, shredded
Salt
Black pepper

Directions:

1. Debone thighs and set the oven to 400 F. Use pepper and salt to season chicken and line a baking sheet with foil.
2. Place chicken onto baking sheet and bake for 40 minutes.
3. Chop bacon, heat skillet and cook bacon for 4-5 minutes until crisp; add peppers and cook for 3 minutes until softened.
4. Add hot sauce, mayo and cream cheese to pot; season with pepper and salt to taste and mix together.
5. Take chicken from oven, cool and remove skin. Transfer chicken to a baking dish and top with cream cheese and bacon mixture. Sprinkle mozzarella and cheddar all over casserole.
6. Bake for 15 minutes and broil for 5 minutes.
7. Spoon onto plates and serve.

(Calories 740 | Total Fats 61.2g | Net Carbs: 2.5g | Protein 31.8g)

Roasted Turkey Legs

(Total Time: 1 HR 5 MIN| **Serve:** 4)

Ingredients:

2 lbs turkey legs
2 tsp Salt
¼ tsp cayenne pepper
½ tsp garlic powder
½ tsp ancho chili powder
1 tsp worcestershire sauce
2 tbsp duck fat
½ tsp black pepper
½ tsp onion powder
½ tsp thyme, dried
1 tsp liquid smoke

Directions:

1. Add all dry spices to a bowl and combine then add wet ingredients and combine thoroughly.
2. Pat turkey legs with paper towel and use seasoning to rub turkey legs.
3. Set oven to 350 F. Heat a cast iron pan and heat fat until it gets smoky, then add turkey legs and sear for 2 minutes on each side.
4. Transfer cast iron pot to oven and roast for 60 minutes, turning halfway through cooking time.
5. Serve hot.

(Calories 382 | Total Fats 22.5g | Net Carbs: 0.8g | Protein 44g)

Asian Grilled Chicken

(Total Time: 55 MIN| **Serve:** 4)

Ingredients:

1 tbsp olive oil

1 tbsp rice wine vinegar

1 tsp garlic, diced

¼ tsp xanthan gum

1 tsp red pepper flakes

6 chicken thighs, with skin and bones

1 tbsp ketchup, low sugar

2 tsp sriracha

1 tsp ginger, diced

4 cups spinach

Salt

Black pepper

Directions:

1. Set oven to 425 F.
2. Rinse chicken and use hand towels to dry chicken and season with black pepper and salt.
3. Combine all ingredients for sauce and coat chicken in sauce. Line a baking sheet with foil and place a wire rack onto baking sheet.
4. Add chicken and bake for 50 minutes until skin is slightly charred and crisp.
5. Take chicken from oven and set aside.
6. Add spinach, salt, pepper and red pepper flakes to fat on the baking tray.
7. Mix together and serve with chicken.

(Calories 606 | Total Fats 53.5g | Net Carbs: 1.5g | Protein 28.8g)

Fettuccine Chicken Alfredo

(Total Time: 25 MIN| **Serve:** 2)

Ingredients:

For alfredo sauce:
2 Tbsp butter
4 Tbsp parmesan cheese (grated)
2 garlic cloves
½ cup heavy cream
½ tsp basil (dried)

For Noodles and Chicken:
2 chicken thighs (skinless and boneless)
Salt
1 Tbsp olive oil
1 pack Shirataki Miracle fettuccine noodles
Black pepper

Directions:

1. Melt butter in a skillet and sauté garlic for 2 minutes.
2. Add cream to the pot and cook for 2 minutes then add parmesan cheese and stir.
3. Add basil, pepper, and salt and cook for an additional 5 minutes over a low flame.
4. Pound chicken thighs and season with pepper and salt.
5. Heat oil in a skillet and fry chicken for 7 minutes per side and remove from pot. Use forks to shred chicken.
6. Prepare noodles as directed on package.
7. Drain and add chicken and noodles to alfredo sauce. Heat for 2 minutes and toss.
8. Serve in bowls.

(Calories 585 | Total Fats 51g | Net Carbs: 1g | Protein 25g)

Ethiopian Doro Watt

(Total Time: 8 HR 10 MIN| **S**erve: 8)

Ingredients:

1 garlic clove (diced)
4 Tbsp Ethiopian berbere
1 chicken (separated into portions)
2 onions (diced)
½ cup butter
2 tsp salt
8 eggs (hard boiled)

Directions:

1. Add chopped onions, butter, garlic, salt and berbere to a slow cooker.
2. Set cooker on low and cook for 8 hours or more.
3. Add chicken to slow cooker and cook for an additional 8 minutes until chicken is tender.
4. Serve with boiled eggs.

(Calories 315 | Total Fats 25g | Net Carbs: 4g | Protein 19g)

Buffalo Chicken

(Total Time: 6 HR 5 MIN| **Serve**: 4)

Ingredients:

3 Tbsp butter
6 frozen chicken breasts
1 bottle of your favorite cayenne peppers sauce
1 cup of your favorite garlic sauce

Directions:

1. Put the chicken in the bottom of your Slow Cooker. Pour the hot sauce over chicken and sprinkle garlic sauce over top.
2. Cover the lid and cook on Low for 6 hours.
3. Once ready, add butter, and cook on Low uncovered for one more hour.
4. Serve hot.

(Calories 517 | Total Fats 18g | Net Carbs: 2.2g | Protein 80g)

Curried Coconut Chicken Fingers

(Total Time: 45 MIN| **Serve:** 5)

Ingredients:
24 oz chicken thighs, boneless with skin
½ cup pork rinds, crushed
2 tsp curry powder
¼ tsp garlic powder
Salt
Black pepper
1 Egg
½ cup coconut, shredded, unsweetened
½ tsp coriander
¼ tsp onion powder

For Dipping Sauce:
¼ cup sour cream
1 ½ tsp mango extract
½ tsp garlic powder
¼ tsp cayenne powder
¼ cup mayonnaise
2 tbsp ketchup, sugar-free
1 ½ tsp red pepper flakes
½ tsp ground ginger
7 drops liquid stevia

Directions:
1. Set oven to 400 F.
2. Beat egg in a bowl and slice chicken into strips.
3. Combine spices, pork rind, and coconut in another bowl. Coat the strips with egg and then also with the dry mix.
4. Place onto a lined baking sheet and bake for 15 minutes and turn over; bake for an additional 20 minutes.
5. Combine all ingredients for dipping sauce in a bowl and serve with chicken.

(Calories 494 | Total Fats 39.4g | Net Carbs: 2.1g | Protein 29.4g)

Greek Chicken

(Total Time: 7 HR 10 MIN| Serve: 4)

Ingredients:

4 boneless chicken thighs
3 cloves of garlic, minced
3 Tbsp lemon juice
1 ½ cups hot water
2 cubes chicken bouillon
3 Tbsp Greek rub

Directions:

1. Coat the slow cooker with cooking spray
2. Season the chicken with the Greek rub, followed by the minced garlic.
3. Transfer the chicken to the slow cooker and sprinkle with lemon juice on top.
4. Crumble the chicken cubes and put in the slow cooker. Pour the water and stir.
5. Cover and cook on low for 6-7 hours.
6. Uncover and serve with a fresh salad.

(Calories 140 | Total Fats 5.7g | Net Carbs: 2.2g | Protein 18.6g)

Chicken Satay

(Total Time: 25 MIN| **S**erve: 3)

Ingredients:

1 lb. ground chicken
4 Tbsp low-sodium soy sauce
3 Tbsp all-natural peanut butter
1 Tbsp lime juice
¼ tsp cayenne pepper
¼ tsp smoked paprika
1 Tbsp rice vinegar
1 Tbsp liquid stevia
2 tsp chili paste
1 clove of garlic minced
2 tsp sesame oil
2 green onions, chopped
1/3 bell pepper, chopped

Directions:

1. Drizzle the sesame oil into a pan over the medium-highheat.
2. Add the ground chicken and the rest of the ingredients and mix well. Cook, stirring occasionally, until the chicken is done.
3. Serve with the green onions and bell pepper on top.

(Calories 393 | Total Fats 23g | Net Carbs: 3.7g | Protein 35g)

Sage and Orange Glazed Duck

(Total Time: 25 MIN| Serve: 1)

Ingredients:

2 Tbsp butter

1 Tbsp swerve

¼ tsp sage

6 oz duck breast

1 tbsp heavy cream

½ tsp orange extract

1 cup spinach

Directions:

1. Use a knife to score the skin of the duck and season with black pepper and salt.
2. Add Sserve and butter to a pot and cook until slightly golden, then add orange extract and sage. Cook until butter has darkened.
3. In another pot, place chicken breast with skin side down and place over a medium heat and cook until skin is crisp.
4. Flip over and add cream to sage mixture before pouring over duck. Cook until duck is done.
5. Add spinach to the pot and cook until wilted.
6. Spoon onto individual plates and serve.

(Calories 798 | Total Fats 71g | Net Carbs: 0g | Protein 36g)

Pad Thai

(Total Time: 30 MIN| Serve: 4)

Ingredients:

3 boneless and skinless chicken thighs

2 packs konjac yam noodles (Shirataki)

2 organic eggs

¼ cup cilantro, chopped

½ cup mung bean sprouts

3 green onions, chopped

2 Tbsp peanuts, chopped

4 Tbsp melted coconut oil

For the sauce:

4 Tbsp lime juice

2 cloves of garlic, minced

1 Tbsp all-natural peanut butter

½ tsp Worcestershire sauce

1½ Tbsp low-sugar ketchup

3 Tbsp fish sauce

1 ½ Tbsp sambal oelek

1 tsp rice wine vinegar

7 drops liquid stevia

Directions:

1. Whisk all the ingredients of the sauce in the bowl. Set aside.
2. Soak the noodles in boiling water for 5 minutes and then dry using a clean towel cloth.
3. Heat the coconut oil in a pan over medium-high. When the pan is hot, sear the chicken on both sides. Set aside and allow the chicken to rest for a few minutes.
4. Using the same pan, throw in the noodles and fry for 6-8 minutes. Crack the eggs on top and scramble with the noodles.
5. Add the sauce to the pan along with the cilantro, mung bean sprouts, and green onions and cook for another 7-10 minutes.
6. Garnish with the chopped peanuts on top.

(Calories 310 | Total Fats 14.9g | Net Carbs: 3.8g | Protein 39.3g)

Creamy Tarragon Chicken

(Total Time: 25 MIN| Serve: 1)

Ingredients:

5 oz chicken breast
¼ onion, sliced
½ cup chicken broth
1 tsp grain mustard
Salt
1 tbsp olive oil
3 oz mushrooms
¼ cup heavy cream
½ tsp tarragon, dried
Black pepper

Directions:

1. Cube chicken and season with pepper and salt.
2. Heat oil in a pan and sauté chicken for 6 minutes, until golden all over. Take from pan and set aside.
3. Add mushrooms and cook for 3 minutes until golden, then add onion and cook for 3 minutes, until soft and translucent.
4. Add broth and bring to a boil for 4 minutes, then add remaining ingredients and adjust black pepper and salt to taste.
5. Return chicken to sauce in the pan and cook for 5 minutes.
6. Serve.

(Calories 490 | Total Fats 40g | Net Carbs: 5g | Protein 32g)

Chicken & Endive Casserole

(Total Time: 40 MIN| **Serve:** 6)

Ingredients:

1 endive head, cut into wide strips
1 1/2 lbs. skinless boneless chicken thighs
1 Tbsp dried oregano
2 cups chopped onions
4 celery stalks, chopped
4 garlic cloves, chopped
1 cup diced tomatoes in juice
2 Tbsp olive oil
8 cups water

Directions:

1. In a large saucepan, heat oil over medium-high heat.
2. Sprinkle the chicken with salt, pepper, and oregano. Add chicken intothe saucepan. Mix in onions, celery, and garlic. Sauté until vegetables begin to soften, about 4-5minutes.
3. Stir in tomatoes. Add broth before bringing to the boil. Reduce heat to medium; simmer until vegetables and chicken are tender, about 15 minutes.
4. Add endive hearts; simmer until wilted, about 3 minutes. Season with salt and pepper.
5. Ladle into bowls and serve hot.

(Calories 144 | Total Fats 7g | Net Carbs: 9g | Protein 9.8g)

Creamy Smoked Turkey Salad with Almonds

(Total Time: 10 MIN| Serve: 4)

Ingredients:

Salad ingredients:
2 cups diced, cooked smoked turkey breast
1/4 cup sliced almonds
1/2 cup diced celery
1/4 cup sliced green onions
1/4 cup shredded cabbage

Dressing ingredients:
4 oz. mayonnaise
2 oz. sour cream
2 drops sweet liquid Splenda
1 tsp curry powder
Salt and pepper to taste

Directions:

1. In a bowl, combine sour cream and mayonnaise and whisk until smooth.
2. Add the spices and continue to whisk until smooth.
3. In a big bowl, combine all salad ingredients and the dressing and toss well.
4. Serve and enjoy.

(Calories 235 | Total Fats 17g | Net Carbs: 10.9g | Protein 9.8g)

Creamy Chicken Salad

(Total Time: 10 MIN| Serve: 4)

Ingredients:

Salad ingredients:

2 cups diced, cooked chicken

1/2 cup sliced green onion

1/4 cup parsley, chopped

1/2 cup diced celery

Dressing ingredients:

4 oz. mayonnaise

2 oz. blue cream cheese softened

1 tsp dried tarragon

1/2 tsp dried thyme

Salt and pepper to taste

Directions:

1. In a bowl, whisk cream cheese and mayonnaise until smooth.
2. Add the herbs and salt and pepper and continue to whisk.
3. Combine the salad ingredients and add dressing to taste, mixing to coat all the ingredients.
4. Serve immediately.

(Calories 250 | Total Fats 12g | Net Carbs: 9.7g | Protein 24g)

Duck Breast with Balsamic Vinegar

(Total Time: 3 HR 25 MIN| **Serve:** 4)

Ingredients:

1 lb. duck breasts
4 Tbsp duck fat (or lark)
4 green onions (chopped)
1 tsp fresh ginger grated
1/2 Tbsp lime juice
Marjoram to taste
2 Tbsp coconut oil
2 Tbsp apple cider vinegar
Salt and freshly ground pepper to taste

Directions:

1. In a frying pan, add 1 Tbsp coconut oil and the duck breast. Sauté on high for about 3-4 minutes.
2. In a deep saucepan, add the duck fat the duck meat. Cook for about 3 hours. Add the chopped green onions in the last 30 minutes of the cooking process.
3. Remove green onion and duck breast from the heat and place them in a separate dish to cool down. Sprinkle the marjoram, balsamic vinegar, and the lime juice over the duck breast.
4. Serve hot.

(Calories 471 | Total Fats 46g | Net Carbs: 2.7g | Protein 10g)

Zesty Herbed Chicken

(Total Time: 20 MIN| Serve: 2)

Ingredients:

2 boneless chicken thighs
2 Tbsp fresh parsley, chopped
½ tsp dried oregano
4 Tbsp lemon juice
1 Tbsp olive oil
Salt and pepper to taste

Directions:

1. Sprinkle the lemon juice on the chicken and season with salt and pepper.
2. Heat the olive oil in a cast iron skillet over medium-high heat and then add the chicken thighs. Cook for 4-5 minutes on each side.
3. Season with oregano and turn of the heat.
4. Transfer the chicken to a serving plate and garnish with fresh parsley on top.

(Calories 469 | Total Fats 22.9g | Net Carbs: 1.2g | Protein 61.1g)

Chicken Pesto Salad

(Total Time: 10 MIN| **Serve:** 6)

Ingredients:

2 cups cooked chicken, chopped
2 Tbsp organic pesto sauce
¼ cup mayonnaise
1 pc celery, chopped
½ onion, chopped
2 Tbsp fresh parsley, chopped
Salt and pepper to taste
Lettuce leaves to serve

Directions:

1. Combine the chicken, pesto sauce and mayonnaise in a bowl. Stir well.
2. Throw in the celery, onion and parsley, season with salt and pepper, and mix well.
3. Serve spooned onto a fresh lettuce leaf on individual plates.

(Calories 406 | Total Fats 20.6g | Net Carbs: 10.8g | Protein 42.7g)

Hot Peri-Peri Chicken on Green Salad

(Total Time: 15 MIN| **Serve:** 1)

Ingredients:

2 cups baby spinach
½ boneless chicken thighs cut into strips
1 Tbsp hot peri-peri sauce
½ ripe avocado, sliced thin
1 strip of bacon, cooked and crumbled

Directions:

1. Cook the bacon first and then use the same pan to fry the chicken. Place the chicken in the pan and cook for 1 minute on one side and then turn over and cook for 5-6 minutes.
2. Place the baby spinach in a salad bowl and then top with the avocado and cooked chicken strips.
3. Sprinkle with the bacon crumbles and drizzle with the hot peri-peri sauce.

(Calories 325 | Total Fats 22g | Net Carbs: 10.8g | Protein 23.9g)

Mediterranean Chicken

(Total Time: 1 HR 10 MIN| **Serve**: 2)

Ingredients:

1 whole free-range chicken, chopped into pieces
1 tsp capers, chopped
4 ripe tomatoes, chopped
½ cup olives, chopped
½ tsp red pepper flakes
Salt and pepper to taste
2 Tbsp olive oil

Directions:

1. Set the oven at 350 F.
2. In a large baking dish, combine the capers, tomatoes, olives, pepper flakes and olive oil. Season with salt and pepper and stir.
3. Add the chicken at the center and place in the oven to cook for an hour.
4. Serve warm.

(Calories 205 | Total Fats 18.2g | Net Carbs: 12g | Protein 2.5g)

Turkey Meatballs

(Total Time: 40 MIN| **Serve:** 2)

Ingredients:

1 lbs. turkey, ground
1 organic egg
3 oz mozzarella cheese, cubed
1 green onion, chopped
2 sun-dried tomatoes, chopped
2 clove of garlic, minced
1 Tbsp fresh cilantro, chopped
½ tsp cumin powder
1 shallot, chopped
Salt and pepper to taste

Directions:

1. Set the oven to 350 F.
2. In a bowl, combine the ground turkey, green onions, sun-dried tomatoes, minced garlic, cilantro, cumin, and shallots. Season with salt and pepper. Combine the ingredients using your hands.
3. Form the mixture into meatballs and flatten them to create patties. Place a mozzarella cube at the center of the patty and form again into a ball.
4. Transfer the meatballs to a baking sheet lined with parchment paper and place in the oven to bake for 30 minutes.
5. Serve warm.

(Calories 509 | Total Fats 19.1g | Net Carbs: 1.8g | Protein 78.7g)

Roast Chicken and Pepper Salad

(Total Time: 40 MIN| **Serve:** 4)

Ingredients:

1.5 lbs. boneless chicken thighs
1 onion, roughly chopped
1 large bell pepper, cut in half and seeded
¼ cup cilantro leaves
1 romaine lettuce
For the dressing
1 Tbsp lime juice
¼ cup mayonnaise
¼ cup sour cream
2 Tbsp olive oil
Salt and pepper to taste

Directions:

1. Set oven to 350 F.
2. Lay the chicken thighs and onions on a baking sheet lined with greased foil .
3. Drizzle with olive oil and season with salt and pepper.
4. Place the chicken in the oven to bake for 20 minutes. When done baking, remove from the oven and let it sit for 10 minutes.
5. Char the bell peppers while waiting for the chicken to bake. Slice into strips when done with the grilling.
6. In a salad bowl, whisk together the ingredients for the dressing. Add the lettuce into the bowl.
7. Top the salad with the cubed baked chicken with onions, and bell pepper on top.
8. Serve immediately.

(Calories 349 | Total Fats 16g | Net Carbs: 7g | Protein 42g)

Chicken and Cucumber Salad

(Total Time: 20 MIN| **Serve:** 2)

Ingredients:

1 cucumber, sliced thinly using a mandolin
2 boneless chicken thighs
1 small green apple, chopped
½ onion, chopped
2 Tbsp organic butter
¾ cup mayonnaise
2 Tbsp mustard
½ tsp oregano, dried
¼ tsp cayenne pepper
Salt and pepper to taste

Directions:

1. Melt the butter in a non-stick pan over medium heat.
2. Add the onions to the pan and sauté for 5-6 minutes. Set aside.
3. Season the chicken with salt and pepper and cook in the same pan. Allow the chicken to rest for at least 3 minutes, before cutting into cubes. Place in the fridge to chill for 30 minutes.
4. Add the mayo, dried oregano, and cayenne into a salad bowl and whisk together. Add the chicken cubes, sautéed onions, cucumber slices, and apples into the bowl and toss together.
5. Serve immediately.

(Calories 502 | Total Fats 41g | Net Carbs: 12g | Protein 19g)

Baked Chicken and Avocado

(Total Time: 30 MIN| **Serve:** 6)

Ingredients:

8 chicken fillets, precooked and shredded
2 large ripe avocados cut thin
1 onion, cut into strips
1 bell pepper, cut into strips
1 cup sour cream
1 cup cheddar cheese
1 Tbsp Sriracha sauce
Salt and pepper to taste

Directions:

1. Set oven to 350 F.
2. Grease a baking dish and lay the avocado slices on top. Set aside.
3. Sauté the onion and bell pepper in a pan until they caramelize.
4. Place the shredded chicken in a bowl and add the rest of the ingredients, including the caramelized veggies (except the avocado slices).
5. Scoop the mixture on top of the avocado slices and then place in the oven to bake for 20 minutes.
6. Serve warm.

(Calories 549| Total Fats 40g | Net Carbs: 13g | Protein 39g)

Crunchy Chicken Waldorf salad

(Total Time: 25 MIN| Serve: 2)

Ingredients:

5 oz full cream plain yogurt

1Tbsp Mayonnaise

2 tsp lemon juice

1/4 tsp salt

1.7 oz chopped cooked chicken breast

½ medium green apple, finely diced

1 cup finely sliced celery

1/2 cup chopped walnuts, toasted

Directions:

1. Whisk mayonnaise, yogurt, lemon juice and salt in a large bowl.
2. Add chicken, apple, celery and 1/4 cup walnuts.
3. Stir to coat well.
4. Serve topped with the remaining 1/4 cup walnuts.

(Calories 169 | Total Fats 11.3g | Net Carbs: 9.6g | Protein 8.6g)

Spicy Chicken Thighs

(Total Time: 60 MIN| **Serve: 8**)

Ingredients:

2 lb. chicken thighs
¼ cup ghee or olive oil
½ tsp garlic powder
½ tsp paprika
½ tsp cumin, ground
¼ tsp cayenne
¼ tsp coriander, ground
1/8 tsp cinnamon, ground
1/8 tsp ginger powder
1 tsp salt
1 tsp yellow curry

Directions:

1. Preheat oven to 425 F.
2. In a small bowl, mix all the spices to create a dry rub.
3. Pat dry the chicken using a kitchen paper towel and place on a baking sheet lined with greased parchment paper.
4. Generously brush the chicken with ghee or olive oil.
5. Rub the spices on the chicken thighs, making sure that you cover every side.
6. Place the chicken in the oven to cook for 50 minutes.
7. Let it cool before serving.

(Calories 227 | Total Fats 20g | Net Carbs: 6g | Protein 21g)

Blackberry and Grilled Chicken Salad

(Total Time: 1 HR 10 MIN| Serve: 2)

Ingredients:

Lemon juice
¼ cup olive oil (extra virgin)
½ cup canned artichoke hearts
¼ cup green olives
1 Tbsp blackberry vinegar
¼ tsp salt
2 chicken breasts (skinless)
1 tsp thyme
7.1 oz lettuce
¼ cup black olives
1 cup blackberries

Directions:

1. Combine thyme, lemon juice, and salt to taste. Coat chicken with half of oil, following it with thyme mixture; put aside for 30 minutes.
2. Set oven to 400 F.
3. Bake for 30 minutes, cool and slice.
4. Rinse lettuce and drain and place in a bowl. Drain artichokes and chop then add to lettuce along with the chicken.
5. Add olives and blackberries and drizzle with leftover oil and vinegar.
6. Serve in individual bowls.

(Calories 587 | Total Fats 39.3g | Net Carbs: 14.6g | Protein 45.2g)

Chili and Lime Meatballs

(Total Time: 25 MIN| **Serve:** 3)

Ingredients:

For meatballs:
2 Tbsp flaxseed meal
2 spring onions, chopped
2 Tbsp cilantro, chopped
½ tsp salt
½ lime juice
1 lb ground chicken
2 Tbsp almond flour
½ red bell pepper, chopped
½ tsp garlic powder
½ tsp red pepper flakes
2 oz cheddar cheese, shredded

For Guacamole:
1 avocado
¼ tsp garlic powder
Salt
½ lime juice
Black pepper

Directions:

1. Set oven to 350 F.
2. Combine chicken, vegetables, cheese, cilantro, and spices in a bowl and add zest.
3. Add flaxseed meal and almond flour and mix together.
4. Roll mixture into balls and place onto a baking sheet greased with cooking spray.
5. Bake for 15 minutes, or until thoroughly cooked.
6. Combine ingredients for guacamole and serve with meatballs.

(Calories 428 | Total Fats 31.3g | Net Carbs: 4.7g | Protein 33.7g)

Sour Avocado and Chicken Moussaka

(Total Time: 35 MIN| Serve: 8)

Ingredients:

8 chicken thighs, cooked
1 cup sour cream
1 cup parmesan cheese
4 avocados
1 onion
1 green pepper
1 Tbsp cayenne pepper sauce
Salt and ground pepper to taste
Coconut oil for greasing

Directions:

1. Preheat oven to 350 F. Grease a baking dish with coconut oil.
2. In a pot, cook your chicken thighs for about 35 minutes. Peel avocados, cut in half and slice into thin strips.
3. Line the bottom of your baking dish with avocado slices. In a small pan, fry chopped peppers and onions until caramelized.
4. Add the chicken into a large bowl and chop it. Add remaining ingredients and mix well.
5. Spoon mixture over the avocado slices. Bake for 20 minutes.
6. Serve hot.

(Calories 345 | Total Fats 25g | Net Carbs: 11g | Protein 20g)

Chicken, Bacon and Avocado Sandwich

(Total Time: 40 MIN| Serve: 2)

Ingredients:

For Bread:
3 oz cream cheese

¼ tsp salt

3 eggs

1/8 tsp cream of tartar

½ tsp garlic powder

For Filling:
1 tsp sriracha

3 oz chicken

2 grape tomatoes

1 Tbsp mayonnaise

2 bacon slices

2 Pepper Jack cheese slices

¼ avocado, sliced

Directions:

1. Preheat oven to 300 F. Place mozzarella into a microwave safe dish and melt for 1 minute, stirring occasionally.
2. Separate eggs into two bowls, add salt and tartar to egg white and whip until soft peaks form.
3. Add cream cheese to egg yolks and beat until thoroughly combined.
4. Add half of white mixture to cream cheese mixture and fold in, repeat with remaining egg white mixture.
5. Place parchment paper on a baking sheet and spoon batter onto sheet, shape into square and top with garlic; bake for 25 minutes.
6. Season chicken with salt and pepper, heat a skillet and coat with cooking spray. Add bacon and chicken and cook thoroughly.
7. Spread mayonnaise on bread and top with chicken, cheese, avocado, sriracha, and tomatoes.
8. Slice in half and serve.

(Calories 361 | Total Fats 28.3g | Net Carbs: 2g | Protein 22g)

Roasted Lemony Chicken & Prosciutto with Brussels sprouts

(Total Time: 40 MIN| Serve: 6)

Ingredients:

2 lbs. chicken tenderloins

4 oz. prosciutto

12 oz. Brussels sprouts

1/2 cup chicken broth

1 1/2 cups heavy cream

1 tsp minced garlic

1 lemon, quartered and seeded

Ghee or coconut oil for frying

Directions:

1. Preheat oven to 400 degrees F.
2. Cut the Brussels sprouts in half and boil for 5 minutes. Remove from heat and set aside.
3. In a frying pan, add 1/2 cup chicken broth and bring to the boil on medium. After that, add heavy cream, minced garlic, and lemon and let simmer for 5-10 minutes, stirring frequently. Remove from heat and set aside.
4. In a separate frying pan, heat up some ghee and add chicken. Cook on medium-high heat for several minutes, and then add chopped prosciutto and stir until chicken is cooked.
5. In a small casserole dish (9×9), layer from bottom to top: Brussels sprouts, chicken, prosciutto, lemon cream sauce on top.
6. Bake in preheated oven for 20 minutes. Serve hot.

(Calories 333 | Total Fats 16g | Net Carbs: 5.2g | Protein 39g)

Pordenone Cauliflower Lasagna

(Total Time: 1 HR 50 MIN| **Serve:** 10)

Ingredients:

12 chicken thighs
30 oz. chopped cauliflower
6 green onions
1 onion, chopped
1 green pepper
6 bacon slices
1 cup cream cheese
1/2 cup heavy cream
8 oz. Pepper Jack cheese, shredded
8 oz. cheddar cheese, shredded
1 Tbsp garlic, minced
Salt and pepper to taste

Directions:

1. Preheat oven to350 F.
2. Chop up a head of cauliflower into florets. Cook the cauliflower in the microwave on the vegetable setting. Set aside.
3. In a pan on the stovetop, toss the chicken thighs with salt and pepper to taste. Add some water to about mid-thigh and cook for 60 minutes. Chop up the onions and peppers and pan fry.
4. Add all of the other ingredients, reserving 2 oz. cheddar and 2 oz. of Pepper Jack cheese.
5. Add the mixture into a large, greased casserole dish and top with the remaining cheese.
6. Cover with foil and cook for 30 minutes. Serve hot.

(Calories 486 | Total Fats 35g | Net Carbs: 13.7g | Protein 28g)

Easy Chicken Cordon Bleu

(Total Time: 50 MIN| Serve: 5)

Ingredients:

1.5 lb. chicken fillet cut in cubes

5.29 oz ham steak, cubed

½ cup Swiss cheese, shredded

½ cup heavy cream ½ cup cream cheese, softened½ tsp garlic powder

Salt and pepper to taste

Directions:

1. Set oven to 350 F.
2. Place the chicken cubes first at the bottom of an oven-safe dish.
3. Season with salt, pepper, and garlic powder.
4. Top with ham cubes and sprinkle with the Swiss cheese on top.
5. Place the cream cheese in the microwave and zap for 10 seconds. Add the heavy cream into the bowl with the melted cream cheese and stir.
6. Pour the cream mixture on top of the dish.
7. Place in the oven to cook for 40 minutes.
8. Serve hot.

(Calories 486 | Total Fats 30g | Net Carbs: 4g | Protein 38g)

"Chicken Alfredo" Pizza

(Total Time: 20 MIN| Serve: 2)

Ingredients:

½ cup leftover chicken, shredded
¾ cup broccoli florets, chopped and steamed
1 cup pizza cheese mix, shredded
1 cup mozzarella cheese, shredded
¼ cup mascarpone cheese
1 Tbsp heavy cream
2 cloves of garlic, minced
Salt and pepper to taste
1 Tbsp garlic infused olive oil
2 Tbsp ghee

Directions:

1. Heat the garlic infused olive oil in a non-stick pan over medium heat.
2. Sprinkle the pizza cheese mix into the pan, allow the cheese to melt, while forming it into a circle (this will be your crust).
3. Add the mozzarella cheese to the pan next and then cook for 5 minutes or until you get a crispy crust. Transfer into a pan and set aside.
4. Using the same pan, add the rest of the ingredients, except the chicken and broccoli, and cook for 5 minutes.
5. Pour half of the prepared Alfredo sauce on top of the pizza crust and set aside.
6. Place the pan back onto the stove and add the steamed broccoli into the pan and stir for a minute.
7. Add the cheesy broccoli on top of the pizza, along with the shredded roasted chicken.
8. Serve immediately.

(Calories 386 | Total Fats 27.8g | Net Carbs: 5g | Protein 29.8g)

Chicken Angel Eggs

(Total Time: 25 MIN| **Serve:** 4)

Ingredients:

1 cup chicken, finely chopped
6 eggs
3 Tbsp mayonnaise
1 Tbsp chopped onion
1/2 tsp dill
1/2 tsp parsley
1 tsp Dijon mustard
1/2 tsp pepper mix seasoning
Old Bay seasoning
Salt and black ground pepper to taste

Directions:

1. In a bowl, mix all the ingredients (except eggs) until well mixed. Refrigerate the chicken salad for 10-15 minutes.
2. Boil your eggs. Shell, cool, and cut in half. Save or toss your yolks.
3. Fill your egg halves with chicken salad. Sprinkle with Old Bay or some other seasoning of your taste. Serve.

(Calories 161 | Total Fats 11g | Net Carbs: 3.7g | Protein 10g)

Oriental Garlicky Chicken Thighs

(Total Time: 1 HR 5 MIN| **Serve:** 4)

Ingredients:

4 chicken thighs
16 whole cloves of garlic
2 Tbsp ghee
2 Tbsp juice of one fresh lemon
1 cup of baby carrots
1 onion, cut into quarters
2 tomatoes cut in half
3 Tbsp garlic olive oil (or extra-virgin olive oil)
Oregano
Salt and pepper

Directions:

1. Preheat oven to 500 F degrees.
2. Grease the bottom of a non-stick frying pan with garlic olive oil (or olive oil). Add the chicken thighs together.
3. In between the thighs, wedge in the garlic cloves, onions, tomatoes and baby carrots.
4. Pour the lemon juice over the chicken thighs. Drizzle with the ghee and garlic oil over the thighs.
5. Sprinkle oregano over the dish and season with salt and pepper to taste.
6. Bake in preheated oven for 25-30 minutes.
7. Reduce heat to 350 degrees and cook for 20 minutes more.
8. Once ready, let cool for 5 minutes on a wire rack and serve hot.

(Calories 237 | Total Fats 14g | Net Carbs: 8.9g | Protein 17g)

Chicken and Broccoli filled Zucchini

(Total Time: 25 MIN| Serve: 2)

Ingredients:

2 Tbsp butter
1 cup broccoli
2 Tbsp sour cream
10 oz zucchini
3 oz cheddar cheese, shredded
6 oz rotisserie chicken, shredded
1 green onion
Salt
Black pepper

Directions:

1. Set oven to 400 F.
2. Slice zucchinis in half lengthwise and use spoons to remove cores. Melt butter and pour equally into each zucchini shell. Add black pepper and salt and bake for 20 minutes.
3. Chop broccoli and place into a bowl with sour cream and chicken. Fill zucchini boats with chicken mixture and top with cheese.
4. Bake for 15 minutes more or until golden.
5. Serve topped with green onion.

(Calories 476.5 | Total Fats 34g | Net Carbs: 5g | Protein 30g)

Baked Creamy Cauliflower-Broccoli Chicken

(Total Time: 1 HR 15 MIN| Serve: 8)

Ingredients:

2 boneless chicken breasts
1 cup chicken broth
3 cups cauliflower
3 cups broccoli, steamed and chopped
2 cups shredded Cheddar cheese
1 cup heavy cream
1 small yellow onion
1/2 Tbsp minced garlic
1 tsp lemon juice
1/2 cup mayonnaise
3 Tbsp ghee
Fresh parsley, chopped
Salt and fresh pepper to taste

Directions:

1. Preheat the oven to 350 degrees F.
2. In a deep saucepot, boil chicken breast until cooked through.
3. Meanwhile, in a frying pan, cook up the garlic and onions on a low heat with the ghee. Add all spices one by one, stirring frequently.
4. While that's cooking, in a food processor blend up your cauliflower.
5. When the onions are soft, add the cauliflower. Cook for 2-3 minutes. Add in the chicken broth. Cook, covered for about 10 minutes.
6. Add the heavy cream and lemon juice and let simmer uncovered on low for about 10 minutes more. At the end, add in mayonnaise and stir.
7. Pull apart your chicken and add half of chicken into the cauliflower cream mixture.
8. Use the other half to line the bottom of an 8x8 casserole dish. On top of the chicken, layer in chopped broccoli.
9. Top with the cauliflower cream mixture.
10. Cover it with cheddar cheese. Bake in preheated oven for 40 minutes. Serve hot.

(Calories 365 | Total Fats 29g | Net Carbs: 9.2g | Protein 17.9g)

Baked Manchego Chicken Wings

(Total Time: 45 MIN| **Serve:** 4)

Ingredients:

20 frozen wings
1 cup of grated Manchego cheese (or Parmesan, Asagio...)
2 Tbsp olive oil
2 tsp dried oregano
1/2 Tbsp garlic powder
1 tsp garlic salt

Directions:

1. Preheat oven to 450 F.
2. In a baking pan greased with olive oil, place frozen chicken wings. Sprinkle with salt and oregano.
3. Bake for 35 minutes.
4. Remove from oven and toss in a bowl with another Tbsp of garlic oil, until well coated.
5. Sprinkle with grated Manchego cheese and garlic powder.
6. Serve hot.

(Calories 446 | Total Fats 33g | Net Carbs: 2.6g | Protein 32g)

Bacon Chicken Patties

(Total Time: 20 MIN| **Serve:** 10)

Ingredients:

12 oz can chicken breast
2 medium bell peppers
¼ cup parmesan cheese
3 Tbsp coconut flour
4 bacon slices
¼ cup sundried tomato pesto
1 egg

Directions:

1. Cook bacon until crisp, put aside until needed.
2. Put bell pepper into a processor and pulse until fine, transfer to a bowl and squeeze out excess liquid.
3. Put bacon and chicken into processor and pulse until thoroughly combined, transfer mixture to bowl with peppers.
4. Add egg, pesto, parmesan and flour to mixture and combine.
5. Heat oil in a skillet and form patties. Add to pan and cook until golden all over.
6. Serve.

(Calories 159 | Total Fats 11.5g | Net Carbs: 1.7g | Protein 9.9g)

Curry-Spiced Salad

(Total Time: 10 MIN| **Serve:** 2)

Ingredients:

2 boneless chicken thighs, cooked and diced
2 celery stalks, diced
¼ cup carrots, minced
¼ cup roasted almonds, chopped
¼ green onions, sliced

For the dressing:
1 tsp curry powder
3 oz. mayonnaise
3 oz. sour cream
¼ tsp stevia
Salt and pepper to taste

Directions:

1. Combine all the ingredients for the dressing, whisk and set aside.
2. Place all the ingredients for the salad in a bowl, drizzle with the prepared dressing, and toss.

(Calories 549 | Total Fats 33.5g | Net Carbs: 17.1g | Protein 45.2g)

Chicken Paprikash

(Total Time: 8 HR 15 MIN| **Serve:** 8)

Ingredients:

3 Tbsp almond or coconut flour
2.2 lbs pounds skinless, boneless chicken breast, butterflied and cut into strips
2 cups chopped onion
1 1/4 cups chicken stock
1 cup chopped red pepper
1/2 cup grated carrot
2 Tbsp sweet paprika
2 Tbsp minced garlic
1 tsp salt
1 tsp freshly ground black pepper
1 punnet mushrooms
1 1/4 cups sour cream or crème Fraiche

Directions:

1. Combine almond flour and chicken in a medium bowl; toss well. Add chicken mixture, chopped onion, and the next 8 ingredients (through mushrooms) to an electric slow cooker. Cover and cook on low for 8 hours.
2. Stir in sour cream and serve.

(Calories 250 | Total Fats 7g | Net Carbs: 5g | Protein 38g)

Chapter 6: Seafood

Sweet and Sour Snapper

(Total Time: 20 MIN| Serve: 2)

Ingredients:

4 fillets snapper
¼ cup fresh coriander, chopped
4 Tbsp juice of lime
6 lychees, sliced
2 Tbsp olive oil
Salt and pepper to taste

Directions:

1. Season the fillets with salt and pepper.
2. Heat the olive oil in a pan over medium heat and cook for 4 minutes on each side.
3. Drizzle the lime juice on the fish; add the coriander, and the sliced lychees.
4. Reduce the heat to low and allow to cook for another 5 minutes.
5. Transfer to a serving plate and enjoy.

(Calories 244 | Total Fats 15.4g | Net Carbs: 0.1g | Protein 27.9g)

Creamy Haddock

(Total Time: 20 MIN| Serve: 2)

Ingredients:

5.3 oz smoked haddock
1/2 boiling water
1 Tbsp butter
¼ cup cream
2 cups spinach

Directions:

1. Heat a saucepan over medium fire.
2. Mix the boiling water with cream and butter in a bowl.
3. Place haddock and sauce in the pan and leave to boil until the water evaporates, leaving a creamy, butter sauce behind.
4. Serve haddock, covered with the sauce on fresh or wilted spinach.

(Calories 281 | Total Fats 10g | Net Carbs: 15g | Protein 18g)

Pan Fried Hake

(Total Time: 15 MIN| Serve: 1)

Ingredients:

1 Tbsp olive oil
Salt and pepper to taste
1 Hake fillet
Fresh lemon wedges

Directions:

1. Heat the olive oil in a large frying pan over medium-high heat.
2. Pat the fish dry with kitchen paper towel and then season with salt and pepper on both sides.
3. Fry the fish for about 4-5 minutes on each side, depending on their thickness, or until they have a golden crust and the flesh flakes away easily with a fork.

(Calories 170 | Total Fats 8g | Net Carbs: 7g | Protein 18g)

Pesto and Almond Salmon

(Total Time: 15 MIN| Serve: 2)

Ingredients:

1 garlic clove
½ lemon
½ tsp parsley
2 Tbsp butter
Handful frisée
1 Tbsp olive oil
¼ cup almonds
½ tsp Himalayan salt
12 oz. salmon filets
½ shallot

Directions:

1. Add almonds, garlic, shallot and olive oil to a processor and pulse until mixture is pasty. Add parsley, salt and squeeze lemon juice into mixture and put aside until needed.
2. Season salmon with pepper and salt.
3. Heat oil in a skillet and place salmon skin side down into pot and cook for 3 minutes per side.
4. Add butter to skillet and heat until melted; coat fish with butter and remove from heat.
5. Serve salmon with frisée and pesto.

(Calories 610 | Total Fats 47g | Net Carbs: 6g | Protein 38g)

Lime Avocado Salmon

(Total Time: 25 MIN| **Serve:** 2)

Ingredients:

1 avocado
2 Tbsp red onions (chopped)
½ cup cauliflower
12 oz. salmon fillets (2)
½ lime

Directions:

1. Place cauliflower in a processor and pulse until texture is similar to rice.
2. Grease skillet with cooking spray and add cauliflower rice to skillet, cook for 8 minutes with the lid on.
3. Add remaining ingredients, except for fish, to a food processor and blend until creamy and smooth.
4. Heat your choice of oil in another skillet and place fillets with skin side down in the pot. Cook for 5 minutes and add pepper and salt to taste. Flip and cook for 5 minutes more.
5. Serve salmon with cauliflower and top with avocado sauce.

(Calories 420 | Total Fats 27g | Net Carbs: 5g | Protein 37g)

Glazed Sesame Ginger Salmon

(Total Time: 40 MIN| Serve: 2)

Ingredients:

2 Tbsp soy sauce

1 Tbsp rice wine vinegar

2 tsp garlic, grated

1 Tbsp ketchup

10 oz salmon fillet

2 tsp sesame oil

1 tsp ginger, diced

1 Tbsp fish sauce

2 Tbsp white wine

Directions:

1. Combine soy sauce, vinegar, garlic, ginger, and fish sauce in a bowl and add salmon. Marinate for 15 minutes.
2. Heat sesame oil in a skillet until smoking, then add fish with skin side down into the pan. Cook for 4 minutes, then flip over and cook for an additional 4 minutes or until done.
3. Remove fish from the skillet and keep warm.
4. Add marinade to the pot and cook for 4 minutes, remove from pot and set aside.
5. Add white and ketchup to the sauce and cook for 5 minutes until reduced.
6. Serve fish with sauce.

(Calories 370 | Total Fats 23.5g | Net Carbs: 2.5g | Protein 33g)

Buttery Shrimp

(Total Time: 25 MIN| **S**erve: 3)

Ingredients:
For battered shrimp:
2 Tbsp almond flour
¼ tsp curry powder
1 egg
3 Tbsp coconut oil
0.5 oz Parmigiano- Reggiano
½ tsp baking powder
1 Tbsp water
12 medium shrimp

For butter sauce:
½ onion, chopped
2 Thai chilies, chopped
½ cup heavy cream
2 Tbsp butter, unsalted
1 garlic clove, diced
2 Tbsp curry leaves
0.3 oz mature cheddar
Salt & Black pepper
1/8 tsp sesame seeds

Directions:

1. Peel and devein shrimp; dry shrimp using a paper towel.
2. Combine all dry ingredients for batter then add water and egg and mix thoroughly to combine.
3. Heat coconut oil in a skillet, dip shrimps into the batter and fry until golden. Take from the pot and put aside to cool.
4. Melt butter in another pot and sauté onion until browned. Add curry leaves, chilies, and garlic and cook for 3 minutes or until aromatic.
5. Lower heat, add cream and cheddar, cook until sauce thickens. Add shrimp and toss to coat.
6. Serve topped with sesame seeds.

(Calories 570 | Total Fats 56.2g | Net Carbs: 18.4g | Protein 4.3g)

Keto Friendly Sushi

(Total Time: 25 MIN| Serve: 3)

Ingredients:

16 oz cauliflower
2 Tbsp rice vinegar, unseasoned
5 sheets nori
½ avocado, sliced
6 oz cream cheese, softened
1 Tbsp soy sauce
Cucumber
5 oz smoked salmon

Directions:

1. Put cauliflower into a food processor and pulse until a rice-like consistency is achieved.
2. Slice each end of cucumber off and slice each side off, throw away center and slice sides into strips. Place in fridge until needed.
3. Heat a skillet and add cauliflower and soy sauce. Cook for 5 minutes or until fully cooked and slightly dried out.
4. Transfer cauliflower to the bowl along with vinegar and cheese, combine and place in refrigerator until chilled. Slice avocados and put aside.
5. Cover bamboo roller with plastic wraps them lay down a sheet of nori, top with cooked cauliflower, salmon, cucumber, and avocados. Roll and slice.
6. Serve.

(Calories 353 | Total Fats 25.7g | Net Carbs: 5.7g | Protein 18.32g)

Stuffed Avocado with Tuna

(Total Time: 20 MIN| **Serve: 4**)

Ingredients:

2 ripe avocados, halved and pitted
1 can (15 oz.) solid white tuna packed in water, drained
2 Tbsp mayonnaise
3 green onions, thinly sliced
1 Tbsp cayenne paprika
1 red bell pepper, chopped
1 Tbsp balsamic vinegar
1 pinch garlic salt and black pepper to taste

Directions:

1. In a bowl, toss together tuna, mayonnaise, cayenne pepper, green onions, red pepper, and balsamic vinegar.
2. Season with pepper and salt, and then pack the avocado halves with the tuna mixture.
3. Ready! Serve and enjoy!

(Calories 233.3| Total Fats 17.77g | Net Carbs: 9.69g | Protein 7.41g)

Herb Baked Salmon Fillets

(Total Time: 35 MIN| **Serve**: 6)

Ingredients:

2 lbs. salmon fillets
1/2 cup chopped fresh mushrooms
1/2 cup chopped green onions
4 oz. butter
4 Tbsp coconut oil
1/2 cup tamari soy sauce
1 tsp minced garlic
1/4 tsp thyme
1/2 tsp rosemary
1/4 tsp tarragon
1/2 tsp ground ginger
1/2 tsp basil
1 tsp oregano leaves

Directions:

1. Preheat oven to 350 degrees F. Line a large baking pan with foil.
2. Cut salmon fillet into pieces. Put the salmon into the Ziploc bag with the tamari sauce, sesame oil, and spices sauce mixture. Refrigerate the salmon and marinade it for 4 hours.
3. Put the salmon in a baking pan and bake fillets for 10-15 minutes.
4. Melt the butter. Add the chopped fresh mushrooms and green onion to it, and mix. Remove the salmon from the oven, and pour the butter mixture over the salmon fillets, making sure each fillet gets covered.
5. Bake for about 10 minutes more. Serve immediately.

(Calories 449 | Total Fats 34g | Net Carbs: 2.7g | Protein 33g)

Salmon with a Walnut Crust

(Total Time: 20 MIN| Serve: 2)

Ingredients:

½ cup walnuts
½ tbsp Dijon mustard
6 oz salmon filets
Salt
2 Tbsp maple syrup, sugar-free
¼ tsp dill
1 Tbsp olive oil

Directions:

1. Set oven to 350 F.
2. Put mustard, syrup, and walnuts into a processor and pulse until mixture is pasty.
3. Heat oil in a pot and place the skin side down in the pan and sear for 3 minutes.
4. Top it with walnut blend and place into a lined baking dish.
5. Bake for 8 minutes.

Place on individual plates and serve.

(Calories 373 | Total Fats 43g | Net Carbs: 3g | Protein 20g)

Baked Glazed Salmon

(Total Time: 30 MIN| Serve: 2)

Ingredients:

2 salmon fillets

For the glaze:
1 Tbsp sweet mustard
1 Tbsp Dijon mustard
1 Tbsp lemon juice
½ tsp chili flakes
1 tsp sage
Salt to taste
1 Tbsp olive oil

Directions:

1. Set the oven at 350 F.
2. In a bowl whisk all the ingredients for the glaze.
3. Place the salmon fillets on a baking sheet lined with parchment paper and brush the salmon fillets with the glaze.
4. Place in the oven to bake for 20 minutes. Serve warm.

(Calories 379 | Total Fats 24.9g | Net Carbs: 4.3g | Protein 35.5g)

Salmon Burgers

(Total Time: 20 MIN| **Serve:** 4)

Ingredients:

1 14.0z can cook salmon flakes in water
2 organic eggs
1 cup gluten-free breadcrumbs
1 small onion, chopped
1 Tbsp fresh parsley, chopped
3 Tbsp mayonnaise
2 tsp lemon juice
Salt to taste
1 Tbsp olive oil
1 Tbsp ghee

Directions:

1. Crack the eggs into a bowl and use a hand mixer to whisk them until fluffy.
2. Add the bread crumbs in the bowl with the egg and combine well.
3. Add the onions, parsley, and mayonnaise and mix again.
4. Add the salmon flakes, and drizzle the lemon juice and olive oil. Season with salt and stir again.
5. Divide the mixture into 4 parts and then create patties using your hands.
6. Heat the ghee in a cast iron skillet over the medium-high fire and fry the patties until golden brown.
7. Serve with a salad on the side.

(Calories 281 | Total Fats 25.2g | Net Carbs: 9.1g | Protein 6.2g)

Keto Crab Sushi

(Total Time: 20 MIN| **Serve:** 1)

Ingredients:

1 ½ cup cauliflower florets, chopped
½ cup softened cream cheese
¾ cup crab meat, cooked
3 Tbsp mayonnaise
1 Tbsp Sriracha
1 nori wrapper

Directions:

1. Pulse the cauliflower florets in a food processor and chop and until you achieve a rice-like texture.
2. Transfer the chopped cauliflower in a microwavable container and zap 5 minutes on high or until the vegetable is cooked.
3. Add the cream cheese with the hot cauliflower and stir. Place the mixture in the fridge and let it cool for an hour.
4. Place the nori wrapper on top of a sushi mat and spread the cauliflower mixture over it. Remember to leave a 1-inch border.
5. Meanwhile, combine all the remaining ingredients in a bowl and then scoop the crab mixture in the middle of the cauliflower rice.
6. Roll the sushi and cut into 6-8 pieces.

(Calories 446 | Total Fats 35.5g | Net Carbs: 23.4g | Protein 10.4g)

Coco Shrimps and Chili Dip

(Total Time: 20 MIN| **Serve:** 2)

Ingredients:

12 large shrimps, peeled and deveined
1 ½ cup coconut shreds, unsweetened
¼ cup coconut flakes
6 Tbsp mayonnaise
3 Tbsp coconut milk
1 egg yolk
Olive oil for frying

For the dip
4 Tbsp mayonnaise
2 tsp chili garlic sauce
1 tsp lime juice

Directions:

1. Pat the shrimp dry and set aside.
2. Combine the coconut shreds, coconut flakes, mayo, coconut milk, and egg yolk. Stir well.
3. Place the shrimps with the coconut mixture. Make sure that the shrimps are well-coated with the mixture.
4. Heat oil in the pan and fry the shrimps until golden brown.
5. Whisk all the ingredients of the dip in a small bowl. Serve alongside with the shrimps.

(Calories 670 | Total Fats 60g | Net Carbs: 7g | Protein 11g)

Tuna/Smoked Salmon Salad

(Total Time: 10 MIN| Serve: 2)

Ingredients:

3.5 oz Smoked Salmon
1 Hard Boiled Egg
½ Avocados
1 cup green beans (Steamed)
5 cherry tomatoes
1 tbsp Red Onion
½ cup celery
Salt and pepper to taste
Drizzle of olive oil to serve

Directions:

1. Place all ingredients into a bowl.
2. Drizzle with olive oil and salt and pepper to taste.
3. Toss lightly and enjoy.

(Calories 270 | Total Fats 14.9g | Net Carbs: 21.6g | Protein 16.7g)

Salmon Salad in Avocado Cups

(Total Time: 35 MIN| Serve: 2)

Ingredients:

1 medium-sized salmon fillet
1 shallot, diced
¼ cup mayo
½ juice of lime
2 tsp fresh dill, chopped
1 Tbsp ghee
1 large avocado, sliced in half and pitted
Salt and pepper to taste

Directions:

1. Preheat oven to 400 F.
2. Place the salmon fillet on a baking sheet and drizzle it with ghee and juice of a lime. Season with salt and pepper and place in the oven to cook for 20-25 minutes.
3. When done, allow the salmon to cook for a few minutes and shred using a fork.
4. Place the salmon in a bowl, add the diced shallot, and mix well.
5. Add the dill and mayo to the salmon mixture and combine well. Set aside.
6. Remove the insides of the avocado halves, making sure that the skin is still intact to make cups.
7. Mash the avocado meat in a bowl and then add to the salmon mixture. Combine well.
8. Transfer the avocado and tuna salad back to the avocado cups and serve.

(Calories 463 | Total Fats 35g | Net Carbs: 6.4g | Protein 27g)

Mackerel Salad

(Total Time: 20 MIN| **Serve**: 2)

Ingredients:

2 eggs (organic)
2 cups green beans
1 Tbsp coconut oil
Black pepper
2 mackerel fillets (6.3 oz.)
1 avocado
4 cups mixed greens
¼ tsp Salt

For dressing:
2 tsp lemon juice
1 tsp Dijon mustard
2 Tbsp olive oil (extra-virgin)

Directions:

1. Cook eggs until hard-boiled and then place into a pan with cold water.
2. Fill a pot with water and add salt to taste. Cook beans for 5 minutes until crisp, drain and put aside until needed.
3. Use a knife to make diagonal slices along the skin of mackerel and use pepper and salt to season.
4. Heat coconut oil in a skillet and place mackerel fillets with skin down into the pan. Cook for 5-7 minutes until skin is crisp. Remove skillet from heat and put aside until needed.
5. Prepare the dressing by mixing all the ingredients together. Slice eggs into quarters and rinse greens and drain.
6. Place greens into a bowl and top with mackerel and eggs; drizzle with dressing.
7. Serve.

(Calories 609 | Total Fats 49.9g | Net Carbs: 16.1g | Protein 27.3g)

Crab Cakes

(Total Time: 20 MIN| Serve: 6)

Ingredients:

1 lb crabmeat

¼ cup parsley, chopped

1 tsp jalapeno pepper, seeds removed and chopped

1 tsp fresh lemon juice

½ tsp mustard powder

½ cup mayonnaise

2 Tbsp olive oil

2 green onions, diced

¼ cup cilantro, diced

1 tsp Worcestershire sauce

1 tsp Old Bay seasoning

1 egg

Salt

Directions:

1. Sort crab and remove shell bits, transfer to a bowl and put aside.
2. Add parsley, jalapeno, lemon juice, mustard powder, green onion, cilantro, Worcestershire sauce and Old Bay seasoning. Gently fold mixture so that crab does not fall apart.
3. Add egg to a bowl and beat, then add mayo and combine. Add crab to mayo mixture and place in a strainer. Put a strainer in a bowl and wrap with plastic wrap; place in refrigerator overnight.
4. Remove the strainer from the bowl and discard excess liquid. Shape crab cakes and cover in the refrigerator while oven heats up.
5. Set oven to 200 F.
6. Heat 1 tbsp of oil in skillet and place 3 of crab cakes into the pan. Cook for 3 minutes until golden and firm, then flip and cook for 3 more minutes. Transfer to baking sheet and place in oven. Repeat with leftover crab cakes.
7. Serve.

(Calories 257 | Total Fats 18.5g | Net Carbs: 0.6g | Protein 19.4g)

Shrimp & Avocado Salad

(Total Time: 45 MIN| **S**erve: 2)

Ingredients:

12 oz. shrimp, peel removed and deveined
1 ripe avocado, peeled, cored, and cut into cubes
3 cups baby spinach
1 tomato, chopped
¼ cup green onions, chopped
¼ cup fresh cilantro, chopped

For the marinade:
4 Tbsp olive oil
2 Tbsp lime juice
Salt and pepper to taste
¼ tsp garlic powder
¼ tsp chili powder

Directions:

1. In a bowl, whisk all the ingredients for the marinade.
2. Add the shrimp into the bowl and toss. Allow to marinate for 30 minutes in the fridge.
3. When the shrimps are ready, heat a non-stick pan over medium fire. Throw in the shrimp and cook for 2 minutes on each side.
4. Toss together the avocado cubes, baby spinach, chopped tomatoes, green onions, and cilantro in a bowl.
5. Top with the cooked shrimp and drizzle with an additional 1 Tbsp of olive oil.

(Calories 428 | Total Fats 22.8g | Net Carbs: 15.1g | Protein 42.5g)

Salmon Salad in Avo Cups

(Total Time: 35 MIN| Serve: 2)

Ingredients:

1 medium-sized salmon fillet
1 shallot, diced
¼ cup mayo
½ juice of lime
2 Tbsp fresh dill, chopped
1 Tbsp ghee
1 large avocado, sliced in half and pitted
Salt and pepper to taste

Directions:

1. Preheat oven to 400 F.
2. Place the salmon fillet on a baking sheet and drizzle it with ghee and juice of a lime. Season with salt and pepper and place in the oven to cook for 20-25 minutes.
3. When done, allow the salmon to cook for a few minutes and shred using a fork.
4. Place the salmon in a bowl, add the diced shallot, and mix well.
5. Add the dill and mayo to the salmon mixture and combine well. Set aside.
6. Remove the insides of the avocado halves, making sure that the skin is still intact to make cups.
7. Mash the avocado meat in a bowl and then add to the salmon mixture. Combine well.
8. Transfer the avocado and salmon salad back to the avocado cups and serve.

(Calories 463 | Total Fats 35g | Net Carbs: 6.4g | Protein 27g)

Tuna Avocado Bites

(Total Time: 15 MIN| **S**erve: 12)

Ingredients:

¼ cup mayonnaise
¼ cup parmesan cheese
½ tsp garlic powder
Salt
10 oz canned Tuna, drained
1 avocado, cubed
1/3 cup almond flour
¼ tsp onion powder
½ cup coconut oil

Directions:

1. Combine all ingredients in a bowl except oil and avocado.
2. Add avocado and fold, use hands to form balls and dust with flour.
3. Heat oil in a pot and fry tuna bites until golden all over.
4. Serve.

(Calories 135 | Total Fats 11.8g | Net Carbs: 0.8g | Protein 6.2g)

Thai Fish Curry

(Total Time: 1 HR 20 MIN| **Serve: 8**)

Ingredients:

1 Tbsp coconut oil
½ Tbsp green Thai curry paste (add more if you like a hotter curry)
8-10 spring onions
2 garlic cloves, crushed
1 Thai red chili, deseeded if you like, and thinly sliced
1 tsp turmeric
1/2 cup chicken stock
1½ cups coconut milk
2.5cm piece of fresh ginger, peeled and sliced
2 tsp xylitol
Juice of 1 lime, plus extra to taste
1 tsp fish sauce
1.5 lbs boneless, skinless white fish, such as cod, hake, and halibut cut into large chunks
Freshly ground black pepper
Chopped coriander leaves, to serve

Directions:

1. Fry Spring onions, garlic and chilies, then stir in green Thai Curry Paste and then sprinkle over the turmeric.
2. Add the stock, coconut milk, ginger, xylitol and juice from a fresh lime and season with pepper. Bring to the boil, stirring to dissolve the paste and xylitol, and then pour the mixture into the slow cooker.
3. Cover the cooker with the lid and cook on HIGH for 1 hour until the flavors are well blended. Add the fish sauce, if using, and add a little more xylitol and fresh lime juice, if you like.
4. Switch the cooker to Low. Add the fish, re-cover and cook until the fish is cooked through and flakes easily.
5. Sprinkle with coriander and lime zest and sliced red chilies.

(Calories 312 | Total Fats 15g | Net Carbs: 20g | Protein 24g)

Chapter 7: Meat

Hearty Portobello Burgers

(Total Time: 25 MIN| Serve: 1)

Ingredients:

½ Tbsp coconut oil
1 tsp oregano
2 Portobello mushroom caps
1 garlic clove
Salt
Black pepper
1 Tbsp Dijon mustard
¼ cup cheddar cheese
6 oz beef/bison

Directions:

1. Heat a griddle and combine spices and oil in a bowl.
2. Remove gills from mushrooms and place into marinade until needed.
3. Add beef, cheese, salt, mustard, and pepper in another bowl and mix to combine; form into a patty.
4. Place marinated caps onto the grill and cook for 8 minutes until thoroughly heated. Place patty onto the grill and cook on each side for 5 minutes.
5. Take 'buns' from grill and top with burger and any other toppings you choose.
6. Serve.

(Calories 735 | Total Fats 48g | Net Carbs: 4g | Protein 60g)

Pork and Shrimp Stuffed Peppers

(Total Time: 2 HR 50 MIN| **Serve:** 3)

Ingredients:

1 lb. shrimps, peeled and deveined
1 lb. ground pork
5 bell peppers, chopped into quarters
4 green onions, chopped
2 cloves of garlic, minced
1 organic egg
1 Tbsp low-sodium soy sauce
1 tsp rice vinegar
2 tsp fish sauce
1 tsp five spice
Salt and pepper to taste
1 Tbsp sesame oil

Directions:

1. Add the spices, onions, sesame oil, fish sauce, and egg in a large Ziploc back.
2. Throw the pork and shrimps into the bag and shake.
3. Place in the fridge to marinate for at least 2 hours.
4. Set the oven to 375 F when you're ready to cook
5. Scoop the pork and shrimp mixture onto the bell pepper, place on a baking sheet and cook in the oven for 35 minutes.
6. Turn the tray around and then bake for another 5 minutes.
7. Allow to rest for 5 minutes before serving.

(Calories 91 | Total Fats 4.7g | Net Carbs: 1.5g | Protein 9.9g)

Spiced Beef

(Total **Time:** 25 MIN| **Serve:** 4)

Ingredients:

1 1/2 lbs. ground beef
½ cup red wine
2 cups mushrooms, sliced
1 bunch of broccoli, chopped into florets
2 cups baby spinach
3 Tbsp keto ketchup
2 Tbsp low-sodium soy sauce
2 cloves of garlic, chopped
1 tsp cayenne
2 tsp cumin
½ tsp onion powder
2 tsp ginger, minced
Salt and pepper to taste

Directions:

1. Heat a cast iron skillet and add the ground beef. Brown the beef before adding the minced ginger and chopped garlic. Stir well.
2. Add the broccoli to the pan as well as the spices and mix well.
3. Pour the wine, along with the spinach and mushrooms. Stir and cook until the spinach has wilted.
4. Add the keto ketchup, stir, and serve hot.

(Calories 515 | Total Fats 35g | Net Carbs: 6g | Protein 33.25g)

Sirloin Tip Cut with Cilantro Sauce

(Total Time: 60 MIN| Serve: 3)

Ingredients:

1 lb. sirloin tip cut

For the marinade:
¼ cup low-sodium soy sauce
4 Tbsp lime juice
2 cloves of garlic minced
½ cup cilantro
¼ tsp chili pepper flakes
¼ cup olive oil

For the sauce:
¼ cup olive oil
2 cloves of garlic, minced
1 cup fresh cilantro
2 Tbsp lemon juice
½ tsp coriander
½ tsp cumin
½ tsp salt

Directions:

1. Place all the ingredients for the marinade in a Ziploc bag. Add the beef, shake and then marinate in the fridge for at least 45 minutes.
2. Make the sauce while waiting for the beef to marinate. Add all the ingredients for the paste in a food processor and pulse until you achieve a smooth paste.
3. After marinating, sear the sirloin on a hot cast iron skillet heated over a medium-high heat.
4. Cook for 3-4 minutes on each side.

(Calories 174 | Total Fats 18.7g | Net Carbs: 2.8g | Protein 32.2g)

Bacon Layered Lasagna

(Total Time: 25 MIN| **Serve:** 2)

Ingredients:

8 bacon strips
¼ cup all-natural pizza sauce
¼ lb. ground beef
1 cup mozzarella cheese, shredded
3 Tbsp parmesan cheese, grated
1 tsp Italian seasoning

Directions:

1. Set oven to 350 F.
2. In a pan, brown the beef over medium heat.
3. Drain the fat from the beef when cooked and then sprinkle with the Italian seasoning.
4. Layer 4 strips of bacon on a 9-inch baking dish and then spread half of the pizza sauce on top. Add the half of the ground beef and half of the mozzarella and parmesan and the cover with the remaining pieces of bacon and repeat the process.
5. Place in the oven to bake for 12-15 minutes, or until the cheese has melted.

(Calories 702 | Total Fats 41g | Net Carbs: 10g | Protein 75g)

Macadamia Crusted Lamb Chops

(Total Time: 30 MIN| Serve: 2)

Ingredients:

6 lamb chops
¾ cup macadamia nuts, ground
2 Tbsp fresh rosemary
Salt and pepper to taste
2 Tbsp ghee

Directions:

1. Set oven to 350 F.
2. Season the lamb chops with salt and pepper. Drizzle with ghee on top.
3. Combine the macadamia nuts and rosemary and roll the lamb chops in the mixture.
4. Place the lamb chops on a baking sheet lined with oil and place in the oven to cook for 25 minutes.
5. Serve warm.

(Calories 856 | Total Fats 66g | Net Carbs: 9.1g | Protein 60.3g)

Slow-Cooker Stroganoff

(Total Time: 6 HR 10 MIN| **Serve:** 4)

Ingredients:

1 lb. beef, cut into cubes
16 oz. cream of mushroom soup
1 onion, chopped
2 carrots, sliced
1 bay leaf
1 Tbsp flour
2 Tbsp ghee
Salt and pepper to taste

Directions:

1. Season the beef with salt and pepper and then sprinkle with the flour.
2. In a cast iron skillet, heat the ghee on medium fire and then add the beef, until cooked through.
3. Transfer the beef cubes in a slow cooker and then add the rest of the ingredients. Stir and then cover.
4. Cook on low for 6 hours. Serve warm.

(Calories 345 | Total Fats 16.8g | Net Carbs: 10.8g | Protein 36.1g)

Spicy Mexican Meatballs

(Total Time: 35 MIN| **Serve**:6)

Ingredients:

1 lb ground beef (92% lean)

4 oz white onion, minced

4 oz Monterey Jack cheese with spicy peppers

1 Tbsp butter

3 cloves garlic

1 tsp chili powder

1 tsp ground cumin

1 tsp ground coriander

1 egg

Sea salt and freshly ground pepper to taste

Directions:

1. Preheat oven to 350 degrees F.
2. In a frying pan, sauté onions in butter until translucent. Set aside
3. Shred and mince the Monterey Jack cheese with spicy peppers. Set aside.
4. In a mixing bowl, whisk the egg with ricotta cheese. Add the spices, salt, and pepper and mix.
5. Add onions and minced Monterey Jack cheese with spicy peppers. Mix well.
6. Add beef and mix until all ingredients are combined.
7. Roll the meat mixture into a ball.
8. Place the meatballs on a cookie sheet, and bake about 20 minutes.
9. Serve hot.

(Calories 321.28 | Total Fats 25.25g | Net Carbs: 2.94g | Protein 19.54g)

Bell Peppers Stuffed

(Total Time: 30 MIN| **Serve:** 4)

Ingredients:

1 lb ground beef
2 spring onions, sliced
1 tsp ginger, diced
8 eggs
2 bell peppers, cut in half
2 tsp garlic, diced
Salt
Black pepper

For Sauce:

1½ Tbsp rice wine vinegar
1 Tbsp chili paste
1/3 cup apricot preserves, sugar-free
1 Tbsp ketchup, low sugar
1 Tbsp soy sauce

Directions:

1. Season beef with pepper and salt and start cooking over a medium flame until browned. Add ginger and garlic and stir together.
2. Push beef to one side and put in spring onions, cook for 2 minutes, then stir together with beef. Take from flame and put aside.
3. Add all sauce ingredients to a pan and cook for 3 minutes, then add half to beef.
4. Stir sauce and beef together and use to stuff peppers.
5. Set oven to 350 F and bake for 15 minutes.
6. Top with reserved sauce and serve.

(Calories 470 | Total Fats 35g | Net Carbs: 6.3g | Protein 32.3g)

Keto Burger Patties

(Total Time: 60 MIN| Serve: 4)

Ingredients:

1.1 lbs ground beef
1 small onion, finely chopped
1 Tbsp mayonnaise
1 red pepper, chopped
¼ cup cheese, grated
1 carrot, grated
1 baby marrow, grated
1 tsp ginger, grated
1 tsp crushed garlic
2 eggs
2 Tbsp almond flour
1 tsp parsley, minced
1 tsp coriander
Salt and pepper to taste

Directions:

1. Mix all ingredients together in a bowl.
2. Form the mixture into balls and flatten into patties.
3. Roll the patties in almond flour and leave to the firm in the fridge for around 30 minutes. This will help to keep the patties from falling apart while cooking.
4. When firm, pan fry the patties in coconut oil. Make sure your oil is hot before adding patties to the pan, you need to hear that oil sizzle. If the oil is not hot, the patty will stick to the pan and fall apart while cooking.
5. Take 1 large brown mushroom, rub with olive oil and some crushed garlic, do not salt. And bake in the oven at 360 F for 15-20minutes. Place the cooked burger on top of the mushroom, add grated cheese and melt in the oven for a couple of minutes.
6. Add 1 Tbsp. mayo to the finely diced red onion, lettuce and tomato, and place on top of the burger.

(Calories 340 | Total Fats 28g | Net Carbs: 3g | Protein 17g)

Meatballs in Coconut Broth

(Total Time: 30 MIN| **Serve:** 4)

Ingredients:

For meatballs:

1 lb. ground beef
4 garlic cloves
2 Tbsp almond milk
1 Tbsp coconut oil
½ onion
½ cup almond flour
1 Tbsp Himalayan salt

For broth:

1 cup broth of choice
1 cup coconut milk

Spices:

1 tsp turmeric
1 tsp crushed pepper (red)
Ginger
2 tsp coriander seeds
1 tsp cinnamon
1 blade lemongrass
Lime zest

Directions:

1. Heat oil in a skillet and sauté garlic and onion until aromatic.
2. Mix together almond milk and flour to make a paste, then add beef and salt.
3. Add onions and garlic to mixture and use hands to combine. Form into balls and put aside until needed.
4. Place meatballs in the skillet you used to sauté, arrange around the edge leaving the middle empty.

5. Add spices to the center of the pan while meatballs cook. Stir spices to make sure they do not burn. When meatballs are browned all over pour in broth and coconut milk. Shake pan or gently stir to combine.
6. Add ginger and lemongrass and cook for 15 minutes.
7. Check if meatballs are cooked, if not cook for an additional 5 minutes.
8. Serve.

(Calories 566 | Total Fats 38g | Net Carbs: 4g | Protein 24g)

Sunday's Best Roast Beef

(Total Time: 6 HR 10 MIN| Serve: 4)

Ingredients:

1.5 lb. beef roast
8oz cream of mushroom soup
½ tsp chili powder
1 tsp smoked paprika
Salt and pepper to taste

Directions:

1. Season the beef with chili powder, paprika, salt, and pepper.
2. Place the beef in a slow cooker and pour over the mushroom soup.
3. Cover and cook on low for 6 hours.

(Calories 252 | Total Fats 53.6g | Net Carbs: 6.4g | Protein 15g)

Apple Rosemary Pork Chops

(Total Time: 20 MIN| **Serve:** 2)

Ingredients:

For Pork Chops:
2 Tbsp olive oil
Black pepper
½ apple
4 pork chops
Salt to taste
Paprika
4 rosemary sprigs

For Vinaigrette:
1 Tbsp lemon juice
Salt to taste
2 Tbsp olive oil
2 Tbsp apple cider vinegar
1 Tbsp maple syrup (sugar-free)
Black pepper

Directions:

1. Set oven to 400 F and place cast iron skillet into the oven to be heated.
2. Dry pork chops and season with oil, paprika, pepper, and salt.
3. Place pork into skillet and sear for 2 minutes per side over a high flame.
4. Add rosemary and apple to pork and bake for 10 minutes, until pork is thoroughly cooked.
5. Combine all ingredients for vinaigrette, except oil, then add oil before serving.
6. Serve.

(Calories 485 | Total Fats 41.2g | Net Carbs: 4g | Protein 25g)

Lemon Mustard Pork Loin

(Total Time: 20 MIN| **S**erve: 2)

Ingredients:

For Pork:
1 Tbsp salt
1 tsp paprika
16 oz. pork loins (4)
1 tsp black pepper
1 tsp thyme

For Mustard Sauce:
¼ cup heavy cream
½ lemon
½ cup chicken broth
1 tsp apple cider vinegar
1 Tbsp mustard

Directions:

1. Rinse pork loin and use paper towels to pat dry. Season with salt, thyme, paprika, and pepper.
2. Heat a skillet and sear pork for 3 minutes per side. Remove from skillet and set aside.
3. Use vinegar and broth to deglaze the pan. Add cream and stir to combine.
4. Add mustard and squeeze lemon juice into sauce. Return pork to pot and use the sauce to coat.
5. Cook for 10 minutes until pork is thoroughly cooked.
6. Serve with the desired side dish.

(Calories 480 | Total Fats 30g | Net Carbs: 1g | Protein 46g)

Cheesy Cauliflower and Bacon Casserole

(Total Time: 1 HR 40 MIN| **S**erve: 6)

Ingredients:

For Beef:
1 Tbsp bacon fat
1 tsp cumin
½ tsp chili powder
¼ tsp cayenne pepper
¼ tsp black pepper
1 Tbsp ketchup, low sugar
1 tsp fish sauce
1 lb ground beef
2 tsp garlic
½ tsp paprika
½ tsp salt
¼ tsp onion powder
¼ tsp Mrs. Dash seasoning
1 Tbsp soy sauce

For Casserole:
1 cauliflower head, florets
4 oz cheddar cheese
10 oz bacon, fried and chopped
4 oz cream cheese

Directions:

1. Add all ingredients for ground beef to a bowl, except fish sauce, soy sauce, and ketchup. Use hands to combine, then place in a plastic bag and add fish sauce, soy sauce, and ketchup.
2. Rub together in bag and seal; place into refrigerator for 30 minutes or more.
3. Cook bacon until crisp, remove from pot and chop, save grease for use later.
4. Add beef to grease in a pot and cook until browned all over.

5. Layer cauliflower in a baking dish and top with cooked beef and cream cheese, then add bacon and top with cheddar cheese.
6. Set oven to 350 F. Bake for 50 minutes until golden and cheese has melted.
7. Dish onto individual plates and serve hot.

(Calories 575 | Total Fats 46.3g | Net Carbs: 4.4g | Protein 26.8g)

Seared Ribeye Steak

(Total Time: 20 MIN| Serve: 3)

Ingredients:

2 medium ribeye steaks
Salt
Black pepper
3 Tbsp bacon fat
Salad to serve

Directions:

1. Set oven to 250 F.
2. Place a wire rack on a baking sheet and place steaks on the rack.
3. Use pepper and salt to season steaks and bake until steak's internal temperature is 123°F.
4. Melt fat in a cast iron pan until it is extremely hot, then transfer steaks to pot and sear on both sides.
5. Let steaks sit for a few minutes before slicing.
6. Serve with a salad on the side.

(Calories 430 | Total Fats 31.7g | Net Carbs: 0g | Protein 30.3g)

Poblano Peppers Stuffed with Pork

(Total Time: 30 MIN| **Serve**: 4)

Ingredients:

1 Tbsp bacon fat
½ onion, chopped
7 baby mushrooms, chopped
1 tsp cumin
Salt
1 lb ground pork
4 poblano peppers
1 vine tomato
¼ cup cilantro
1 tsp chili powder
Black pepper

Directions:

1. Slice peppers and remove seeds before placing onto a baking sheet lined with foil and broil for 10 minutes. Turn every 2 minutes to cook evenly.
2. Heat bacon fat in a skillet and cook pork for 10 minutes. Add pepper, chili, salt, and cumin to pork, stir to combine.
3. Add garlic and onion, cook, until soft, then add mushrooms.
4. Add tomatoes and cilantro to the pan and cook for 2 minutes.
5. Set oven to 350 F. Use pork mixtures to fill peppers.
6. Bake for 8 minutesand serve warm.

(Calories 367 | Total Fats 27.3g | Net Carbs: 5g | Protein 21.3g)

Crispy Slow Roasted Pork Shoulder

(Total Time: 12 HR| Serve: 20)

Ingredients:

3 ½ Tbsp salt
1 tsp black pepper
1 tsp onion powder
8 lbs pork shoulder
2 tsp oregano
1 tsp onion powder

Directions:

1. Rinse and dry pork and let it sit at room temperature for a few hours.
2. Set oven to 250 F. Combine seasonings and rub pork all over.
3. Line baking sheet with foil and place a wire rack onto sheets. Place pork shoulder onto rack and bake for 10 hours and remove from oven.
4. Cover with foil and put aside for 15 minutes. Set oven to 500 F and return pork to oven without foil. Bake for 20 minutes, turning every 5 minutes.
5. Remove from oven, cover with foil and let it sit for 20 minutes.
6. Slice and serve.

(Calories 461 | Total Fats 36.7g | Net Carbs: 0.2g | Protein 30.3g)

Italian Style Meatballs

(Total Time: 25 MIN| Serve: 4)

Ingredients:

1 tsp oregano
2 tsp garlic, diced
3 Tbsp tomato paste
2 eggs
½ cup mozzarella cheese
Salt
1 ½ lbs ground beef
½ tsp Italian seasoning
½ tsp onion powder
3 Tbsp flaxseed meal
½ cup olives, sliced
1 tsp Worcestershire sauce
Black pepper
Side salad to serve

Directions:

1. Set oven to 400 F.
2. Add beef to a bowl along with Italian seasoning, onion powder, flaxseed meal, olives, Worcestershire sauce, oregano, garlic, tomato paste, eggs, mozzarella cheese, pepper, and salt.
3. Mix together and form into balls and place onto a baking sheet lined with foil.
4. Bake for 20 minutes.
5. Serve with a salad on the side.

(Calories 594 | Total Fats 44.8g | Net Carbs: 3.8g | Protein 36.8g)

Grilled Asian Short Ribs

(Total Time: 2 HR 15 MIN| Serve: 4)

Ingredients:

For marinade and ribs:
¼ cup soy sauce

2 Tbsp fish sauce

1 ½ lbs short rib

2 Tbsp rice vinegar

For spice rub:
½ tsp onion powder

½ tsp red pepper flakes

¼ tsp cardamom

1 tsp ground ginger

½ tsp garlic, diced

½ tsp sesame seed

1 Tbsp Salt

Directions:

1. Combine all ingredients for marinade in a bowl and place ribs into marinade; put aside for 1-2 hours.
2. Transfer ribs and marinade into a baking dish. Combine spice rub and coat ribs all over.
3. Heat grill and cook for 10 minutes. Alternately, you may place ribs into a grill pan and place into oven for 15 minutes.
4. Serve warm.

(Calories 417 | Total Fats 31.8g | Net Carbs: 0.9g | Protein 29.5g)

Cheeseburger Waffles

(Total Time: 30 MIN| **S**erve: 4)

Ingredients:

For Waffles:

2 eggs
¼ tsp garlic powder
4 Tbsp almond flour
Salt
1.5 oz cheddar cheese
1 cup cauliflower, crumbled
¼ tsp onion powder
3 Tbsp parmesan cheese
Black pepper

For topping:

4 bacon slices, chopped
1.5 oz cheddar cheese, shredded
4 oz ground beef
4 Tbsp BBQ sauce, sugar-free
Salt
Black pepper

Directions:

1. Add crumbled cauliflower to a bowl, along with parmesan, spices, almond flour, half of cheddar cheese and eggs.
2. Heat skillet and cook bacon for 2 minutes, then add beef and cook thoroughly. Transfer any grease from meats into cauliflower mix.
3. Blend the waffle mixture with an immersion blender. Heat waffle iron and pour in mixture.
4. Add BBQ sauce to meat as waffles cook.
5. Transfer waffles to a plate and top with cheese; broil for 2 minutes.
6. Serve warm

(Calories 354 | Total Fats 29.8g | Net Carbs: 3g | Protein 18.8g)

Slow Cooker Beef with Dried Herbs

(Total Time: 8 HR 10 MIN| Serve: 5)

Ingredients:

1 1/2 lbs. lean beef
2 celery ribs
1 cup beef broth
2 Tbsp amaranth flour
2 Tbsp almond butter
2 Tbsp olive oil
1 tsp mustard
2 Tbsp fresh lemon juice
4 Tbsp chopped parsley
Salt, pepper, dried thyme, dried marjoram

Directions:

1. In a bowl, toss the beef with the amaranth flour. Heat the butter and oil in a skillet; add the beef and cook, stirring, until browned.
2. In a slow cooker, combine the browned beef with remaining ingredients, except lemon juice and parsley.
3. Cover and cook on Low for 6 to 8 hours.
4. Once ready, stir in lemon juice and parsley and serve hot.

(Calories 387.96 | Total Fats 12.53g | Net Carbs: 2.56g | Protein 20.96g)

Lamb Cutlets with Garlic Sauce

(Total Time: 40 MIN| Serve: 10)

Ingredients:

4 lbs. lamb cutlets
1 small head of garlic, cloves peeled
2 Tbsp apple cider vinegar
1/2 cup water
1/4 cup extra-virgin olive oil
Pinch salt and black ground pepper to taste

Directions:

1. Crush the garlic cloves thoroughly in a mortar. In a bowl, add the vinegar and water and mix it well with the crushed garlic. Set aside.
2. In a large frying pan, pour the olive oil and fry the lamb cutlets until nicely brown.
3. Add the garlic mixture and let it cook gently for about 10 minutes.
4. Shake the frying pan to spread the garlic mixture evenly over the lamb.
5. Season with salt and black pepper to taste. Serve.

(Calories 416 | Total Fats 28g | Net Carbs: 0.16g | Protein 36g)

Hot Mexican Meatballs

(Total Time: 35 MIN| **Serve:** 6)

Ingredients:

1 lb. ground beef (92% lean)

4 oz. white onion, minced

4 oz. Monterey Jack cheese with spicy peppers

1 Tbsp butter

3 cloves garlic

1 1/2 tsp chili powder

1 tsp ground cumin

1 tsp ground coriander

1 egg

Sea salt and freshly ground pepper to taste

Directions:

1. Preheat oven to 350 degrees F.
2. In a frying pan, sauté onions in butter until translucent. Set aside
3. Shred and mince the Monterey Jack cheese with spicy peppers. Set aside.
4. In a mixing bowl, whisk the egg with ricotta cheese. Add the spices, salt, and pepper and mix.
5. Add onions and minced Monterey Jack cheese with spicy peppers. Mix well.
6. Add beef and mix until all ingredients are combined.
7. Roll the meat mixture into a ball.
8. Place the meatballs on a cookie sheet, and bake about 20 minutes, until well browned.
9. Serve hot.

(Calories 321 | Total Fats 25g | Net Carbs: 2.9g | Protein 19g)

Baked Cheesy Meatballs

(Total Time: 35 MIN| Serve: 6)

Ingredients:

1 lb. ground beef (lean)
2 white onion
1 cup grated Cheddar cheese
4 oz. Gruyere cheese
1 egg
1.5 tsp nutmeg
1.5 tsp allspice
Sea salt and freshly black pepper to taste
Butter for greasing

Directions:

1. Preheat oven to 350 F.
2. In a greased frying pan, sauté onions until translucent. Remove from heat, and let cool.
3. In a food processor, mince the Gruyere cheese. Set aside.
4. In a mixing bowl, whisk the egg with grated Cheddar cheese. Add the spices, salt, and pepper and mix.
5. Add in onions and Gruyere cheese. Mix well until smooth.
6. Add the beef and mix until all ingredients are combined well.
7. Divide meat mixture and roll each piece into a ball.
8. Place the meatballs on a cookie sheet, and bake in preheated oven about 20 minutes andserve hot.

(Calories 385 | Total Fats 29g | Net Carbs: 4.7g | Protein 25g)

Tangy Asian Short Ribs

(Total Time: 20 MIN| Serve: 3)

Ingredients:

1 ½ lb. short ribs

For the rub:
1 tsp ginger, grated
1 clove of garlic, minced
½ tsp onion powder
½ tsp red pepper flakes
¼ tsp cardamom
½ tsp sesame seed
1 tsp salt

For the marinade:
¼ low-sodium soy sauce
2 Tbsp fish sauce
2 Tbsp rice vinegar

Directions:

1. Whisk all the ingredients for the marinade and pour it over the ribs. Allow the ribs to marinate for an hour.
2. Mix all the ingredients for the rubbing
3. Roll marinated ribs in the rubbing mixture and making sure to evenly coat.
4. Heat the grill and cook for 4-5 minutes on each side.

(Calories 417 | Total Fats 31.8g | Net Carbs: 0.9g | Protein 29.5g)

Beanless Chili con Carne

(Total Time: 60 MIN| Serve: 5)

Ingredients:

1 lb ground beef
1 green pepper, chopped
1 onion, chopped
2 Tbsp curry powder
2 Tbsp cumin
1 Tbsp coconut oil
1 tsp onion powder
1 tsp black pepper
1 lb Italian sausage, spicy
1 yellow pepper, chopped
16 oz tomato sauce
2 Tbsp chili powder
1 Tbsp garlic, diced
1 Tbsp butter
1 tsp salt

Directions:

1. Heat oil and butter in a pan, heat thoroughly and add garlic, onions and bell peppers. Cook for 3 minutes then add beef and sausage.
2. Cook for 5 minutes until browned, then add onion and chili powder. Stir to combine and add tomato sauce. Lower flame and cook for 20 minutes.
3. Add cumin and curry, stir and cook for 45 minutes or until chili thickens to your liking.
4. Serve in bowls.

(Calories 415 | Total Fats 25g | Net Carbs: 6g | Protein 146g)

Delicious Meaty Meatloaf

(Total Time: 1 HR 20 MIN| **Serve:** 4)

Ingredients:

7 oz prosciutto, sliced thin
7 oz provolone, sliced thin
2 cups baby spinach
1 cup tomato sauce
½ cup tomato paste
1 Tbsp apple cider vinegar
4 Tbsp stevia
1 lb. ground pork
½ onion, chopped
½ cup bell pepper, chopped
2 cloves of garlic, minced
¼ cup parmesan cheese, grated
2 organic eggs
1 tsp oregano, dried
1 tsp basil, dried
Salt and pepper to taste
1 Tbsp butter

Directions:

1. Set the oven at 350 F.
2. Melt the butter in a pan over medium heat. Throw in the baby spinach and season with salt and pepper. Cook until the leaves wilt.
3. In a bowl, combine the tomato sauce and paste, along with the apple cider and stevia. Stir and set aside.
4. In another bowl, combine the pork, onion, bell pepper, garlic, parmesan, and herbs. Mix well.
5. Lay a parchment paper about 10 inches long and spread the meat on top. Arrange the prosciutto on top, followed by the spinach and provolone to create a meatloaf. Seal sides.
6. Place the meatloaf in a loaf pan lined with foil and pour the tomato sauce on top.
7. Bake in the oven for a little over an hour or until the inner temperature reaches 165 F.

(Calories 516 | Total Fats 37g | Net Carbs: 8g | Protein 37g)

Pulled Pork Shoulder

(Total Time: 5 HR 10 MIN| **Serve:** 4)

Ingredients:

2 lbs. whole pork shoulder
2 tsp paprika
1 tsp salt
1 tsp pepper
½ tsp cumin
¼ tsp cinnamon

Directions:

1. Set the oven at 450 F.
2. Score the skin of the pork with a sharp knife.
3. Combine all of the ingredients of the rub and then smother it over the pork.
4. Place in a baking dish and cook in the oven for 30 minutes.
5. Take out of the oven and cover the dish with foil.
6. Lower the heat to 350 F and place the covered dish in the oven to cook for another 4 hours and 30 minutes.
7. Take the pork out of the oven and pull using forks. Serve with a low-carb BBQ sauce.

(Calories 534 | Total Fats 39g | Net Carbs: 0.9g | Protein 42.4g)

Slow Roast Lamb

(Total Time: 7 HR 15 MIN| Serve: 3)

Ingredients:

1 lb. leg of lamb
2 Tbsp Dijon mustard
3 cloves of garlic
3 sprigs of thyme
½ tsp rosemary, dried
3 mint leaves
1 Tbsp liquid stevia
¼ cup olive oil
Salt and pepper to taste

Directions:

1. Cut large slits on the leg of lamb and place in a slow cooker.
2. Combine the mustard, olive oil and stevia and then rub over the lamb. Season with salt and pepper.
3. Insert the garlic and rosemary into the slits.
4. Cover and cook on low for 7 hours.
5. Add the mint leaves and thyme after 7 hours and cook for another hour.

(Calories 413 | Total Fats 35.2g | Net Carbs: 0.5g | Protein 26g)

Lamb Curry & Spinach

(Total Time: 8 HR 25 MIN| **Serve:** 5)

Ingredients:

1/3 cup coconut or olive oil
3 chopped yellow onions
4 cloves garlic, peeled and minced
2cm piece of ginger, peeled and grated
2 tsp ground cumin
1 ½ tsp cayenne pepper
1½ tsp tround turmeric
2 cups beef stock, high quality
53 oz leg of lamb, cut into 2cm cubes
Salt
6 cups baby spinach
1 1/5 cups plain full-fat yogurt

Directions:

1. Place oil into a large skillet over medium to high heat.
2. Add chopped onions and garlic to the skillet and sauté until brown, 4 - 5 minutes.
3. Then add ginger, cayenne pepper, turmeric, and cumin to the skillet. Stir and let the flavor develop for 30 seconds.
4. Pour in beef stock and scrape the browned bits off the bottom of the skillet.
5. Once the stock comes to a boil, take the skillet off the heat.
6. Place the lamb in your slow cooker. Add the contents of skillet and 1 tsp of salt.
7. Cover the slow cooker with the lid and cook on high for 4 hours, or low for 8 hours.
8. 5 minutes before the slow cooker is done, stir the spinach into the dish and wait for it to wilt.
9. Before serving, stir in the yogurt.
10. Serve and enjoy.

(Calories 304 | Total Fats 16.32g | Net Carbs: 5.5g | Protein 32.85g)

Cheeseburger Casserole

(Total Time: 45 MIN| **Serve**: 6)

Ingredients:

3 bacon slices
1 ¼ cups cauliflower
½ tsp garlic powder
2 Tbsp ketchup, no sugar
2 Tbsp mayonnaise
4 oz cheddar cheese
1 lb ground beef
½ cup almond flour
1 Tbsp psyllium husk powder
½ tsp onion powder
1 Tbsp Dijon mustard
3 eggs
Salt
Black pepper

Directions:

1. Set oven to 350 F.
2. Place cauliflower into a processor and pulse until fine like rice. Add remaining dry ingredients, except for cheese.
3. Add beef and bacon in processor until combined and pasty.
4. Heat skillet and cook meat for 8 minutes, then add to dry ingredients in a bowl, along with half of cheese. Stir to combine and line a baking dish with parchment paper.
5. Press mixture into dish and top with leftover cheese. Bake for 30 minutes on top rack.
6. Take from heat, cool and slice before serving.

(Calories 478 | Total Fats 35.5g | Net Carbs: 3.6g | Protein 32.2g)

Leftover Meat Salad

(Total Time: 10 MIN| **Serve:** 1)

Ingredients:

1 cup left-over meat (chicken or pork), shredded
2 cups iceberg lettuce
1 Tbsp mayonnaise
2 Tbsp sour cream
Salt and pepper to taste

Directions:

1. Whisk the mayo and sour cream in a salad bowl.
2. Add the lettuce to the bowl, along with the shredded meat.
3. Season with salt and pepper and toss.
4. Serve immediately.

(Calories 252 | Total Fats 53.6g | Net Carbs: 6.4g | Protein 15g)

Asian-Flavored Steak

(Total Time: 55 MIN| Serve: 4)

Ingredients:

4 steaks of your choosing

For the glaze marinade:

½ tsp sesame oil

½ tsp chili flakes

1 tsp ginger, grated

½ cup low-sodium soy sauce

2 green onions

Directions:

1. Combine all the ingredients for the marinade in a large bowl and whisk well.
2. Place the steaks in the bowl and marinate for at least 45 minutes.
3. Heat the grill on high and cook the steaks for 5 minutes on each side, or depending on your liking.

(Calories 531 | Total Fats 13.7g | Net Carbs: 4.7g | Protein 94.4g)

Stir Fried Beef

(Total **Time:** 25 MIN| **Serve:** 2)

Ingredients:

1 Tbsp olive oil
12 oz sirloin steak, cut into strips
1 onion, chopped
2 cloves of garlic, crushed
1 cup cherry tomatoes, quartered
1 red bell pepper chopped
2 tsp ginger, grated
4 Tbsp organic apple cider vinegar
Salt and pepper to taste

Directions:

1. Drizzle the olive oil on a non-stick pan and warm over medium heat.
2. Season the sirloin with salt and pepper and sear in the hot oil for 4 minutes on each side.
3. While waiting, whisk the ginger and apple cider together and pour over the steak in the pan.
4. Add the chopped onion, garlic, bell pepper, and cherry tomatoes with the beef and reduce the heat to low.
5. Cover the pan and allow to simmer for 5 minutes.
6. Turn off the heat and then allow the beef to rest for 5 minutes before serving.

(Calories 359 | Total Fats 19g | Net Carbs: 10g | Protein 39)

Pizza on Lettuce Rolls

(Total Time: 15 MIN| Serve: 2)

Ingredients:

6 romaine lettuce leaves

3 Tbsp mayonnaise

6 slices of provolone cheese

6 slices salami

6 slices pepperoni

6 slice ham

Directions:

1. Lay the lettuce leaves on a serving plate.
2. Spread the mayonnaise on top of the leaves and layer with the cheese, salami, pepperoni, and ham.
3. Carefully roll the leaves and secure with a toothpick.
4. Serve immediately.

(Calories 592 | Total Fats 46g | Net Carbs: 6g | Protein 37g)

Spicy Bacon-Wrapped Dogs

(Total Time: 15 MIN| **Serve:** 2)

Ingredients:

1 Tbsp ghee
1 onion, chopped
1 red bell pepper, chopped
1 pc jalapeno, seeds removed and chopped
4 beef hot dogs
4 bacon strips
3 cheddar cheese slices

Directions:

1. Heat the ghee in a non-stick pan over medium heat.
2. Add the onions, bell peppers, and chopped jalapeno and sauté for 4 minutes. Remove from the pan and set aside.
3. Wrap the hotdog with bacon strips and secure with a toothpick. Cook in the same pan where the peppers were cooked.
4. Fry the dogs for 5 minutes, or until crispy on both sides.
5. Lay the cheese slices on top of the cooking hotdogs and cover for 30 seconds to cook, or until the cheese melts.
6. Serve the hot dogs with the sautéed peppers on the side.

(Calories 349 | Total Fats 29g | Net Carbs: 8g | Protein 14g)

Spring Roll in a Bowl

(Total Time: 25 MIN| Serve: 12)

Ingredients:

1.1 lbs pork mince
2 cups cabbage, shredded finely
2 cup grated carrot
2 cups grated baby marrows
1 cup mushrooms
4 Tbsp coconut oil
1/2 cup soya sauce
1 cup chicken stock
2 tsp vinegar
5 cloves garlic, minced
4 tsp grated ginger
4 finely sliced spring onions
½ cup toasted sesame seeds
1 hard-boiled egg, chopped

Directions:

1. Heat the coconut oil and fry the garlic, spring onions and ginger.
2. Add the pork mince and brown.
3. Add the cabbage and carrot to the pot and toss to combine. Stir in the soy sauce.
4. Cover and cook until the vegetables are soft, about 15 minutes.
5. Dish up and add chopped hard-boiled egg over each of the bowls.
6. Garnish with sesame seeds once you have dished up.

(Calories 219 | Total Fats 9.7g | Net Carbs: 32.6g | Protein 3.2g)

Homemade Meatballs

(Total Time: 25 MIN| Serve: 12)

Ingredients:

1.1 lbs ground beef
1 whole egg
½ cup almond flour
2 cloves of garlic, minced
1 tsp oregano, dried
1 tsp thyme, dried
1 cup mozzarella cheese, shredded
Salt and pepper to taste
½ cup homemade marinara sauce

Directions:

1. Preheat oven to 450 F.
2. In a large bowl, place the ground beef, egg, almond flour, garlic, oregano, thyme, and season with salt and pepper. Also, add the cheese.
3. Using your hands, mix all the ingredients together, making sure that everything is well combined.
4. Create 25 meatballs and lay them on a baking sheet lined with parchment paper.
5. Cook in the oven to cook for 15 minutes or until golden brown.
6. Serve the meatballs with marinara sauce.

(Calories 117 | Total Fats 9.3g | Net Carbs: 0.9g | Protein 7g)

Beef Shred Salad

(Total Time: 10 MIN| **S**erve: 2)

Ingredients:

2 cups beef, shredded
1 yellow pepper, sliced thinly lengthwise
1 white onion, sliced lengthwise
6 butter lettuce
2 tsp mayo
1/8 tsp chili flakes

Directions:

1. Place the butter lettuce on a serving plate. Spread mayo on the lettuce and top with the shredded beef.
2. Place pepper slices and onions on top and season with chili flakes.
3. Serve as it is, or rolled up.

(Calories 338 | Total Fats 25g | Net Carbs: 2.4g | Protein 24g)

Cheesy Hotdog Pockets

(Total Time: 50 MIN| Serve: 2)

Ingredients:

2 beef hot dogs
2 thick sticks of quick-melt cheese (or mozzarella)
4 slices of bacon
1/8 tsp garlic powder
1/8 tsp onion powder
Salt and pepper to taste

Directions:

1. Preheat oven to 400 F.
2. Cut the hotdogs lengthwise to create slits.
3. Insert the cheese sticks in the hotdog and then wrap the bacon around the beef hot dog. Secure the bacon using a toothpick.
4. Transfer the hotdogs on a baking sheet lined with foil and flavor with garlic and onion powder.
5. Place in the oven to cook for 40 minutes, or until the hotdogs turns golden brown and the cheese is melted.
6. Serve with a veggie salad on the side.

(Calories 378 | Total Fats 35g | Net Carbs: 0.3g | Protein 17g)

Cheese Steak Salad

(Total Time: 35 MIN| Serve: 2)

Ingredients:

For steaks:
¼ tsp salt
2 Tbsp ghee
10.6 oz ribeye steak

For salad:
2 ½ oz onions (sliced)
1 green pepper (sliced)
½ cup cheddar cheese (grated)
Salt
1 Tbsp ghee
1 garlic clove (diced)
1 red pepper (sliced)
7 oz. mixed greens
Fresh herbs

Directions:

1. Let steaks sit at room temperature for 15 minutes. Pat dry with paper towel and melt ghee. Coat with ghee, pepper, and salt.
2. Heat a cast iron pot and sear steaks for 4 minutes, until browned all over. Lower heat and cook steak until desired doneness have been achieved.
3. Take steaks from pot and put aside to rest for 7 minutes before slicing.
4. Slice vegetables and add ghee to skillet and melt. Cook for 5 minutes, until veggies are crisp.
5. Add lettuce to bowl and top with cooked veggies, steak, and top with cheese.
6. Serve warm.

(Calories 622 | Total Fats 47.1g | Net Carbs: 12.3g | Protein 38.1g)

Sausage and Cheese Balls

(Total Time: 20 MIN| Serve: 12)

Ingredients:

12 cubes cheddar cheese
6 oz. cheddar cheese (shredded)
12 oz. ground sausage

Directions:

1. Combine sausage and cheese in a bowl.
2. Divide mixture into 12 parts.
3. Place cheese in middle of sausage mixture and form into balls.
4. Place on a tray and put into the freezer.
5. Heat oil in a deep pot and fry for 5 minutes.
6. Serve warm.

(Calories 173 | Total Fats 14g | Net Carbs: 1g | Protein 10g)

Bunless Bacon and Almond Butter Burger

(Total Time: 50 MIN| Serve: 4)

Ingredients:
For Almond Sauce:
1 cup water
4 Thai chilis
1 tsp swerve
1 cup almond butter
4 garlic cloves
6 Tbsp coconut amino
1 Tbsp rice vinegar

For Burger:
4 pepper jack cheese slices
1 red onion, sliced
Salt & Black pepper
1 ½ lbs ground beef
8 bacon slices
8 romaine lettuce leaves

Directions:

1. Prepare almond butter sauce by adding water and almond butter to a saucepan.
2. Heat mixture until it starts to thicken, stirring occasionally, then add coconut aminos.
3. Add garlic, vinegar, swerve and peppers. Pulse until thoroughly combined.
4. Transfer pepper mixture to butter sauce in pot and mix together.
5. Put aside until needed.
6. Prepare burgers by seasoning beef with pepper and salt. Shape into patties and make an indent in each.
7. Place patties on baking sheet and put into the broiler for 7 minutes, until golden. Flip patties and broil for an additional 7 minutes.
8. Top with cheese and bake for 5 minutes until melted.
9. Slice onions and cook bacon.
10. Arrange burgers by placing patties onto lettuce and topping with almond sauce, onion and bacon. Serve on individual plates.

(Calories 890 | Total Fats 68g | Net Carbs: 8g | Protein 54.4g)

Pigs in a Blanket

(Total Time: 40 MIN| Serve: 36)

Ingredients:

8 oz cheddar cheese
1 Tbsp psyllium husk powder
1 egg
½ tsp black pepper
37 mini hot dogs
3/ cup almond flour
3 Tbsp cream cheese
½ tsp salt
½ tsp black pepper

Directions:

1. Place mozzarella in a microwave safe dish and heat until cheese melts and is bubbling.
2. Add flour, salt, pepper and husk powder to cheese and mix together until dough is formed.
3. Spread dough on a plate and place into refrigerator for 20 minutes until firm.
4. Set oven to 400 F.
5. Transfer chilled dough to a piece of foil and slice into 37 strips.
6. Wrap each hot dog and place onto baking sheet. Bake for 15 minutes and broil for 2 minutes.
7. Serve warm.

(Calories 72 | Total Fats 5.9g | Net Carbs: 0.6g | Protein 3.8g)

Cheesy Crust Pizza

(Total Time: 35 MIN| Serve: 12)

Ingredients:

½ lb ground beef
2 eggs
1 tsp garlic powder
¼ tsp basil
¼ tsp turmeric
8 oz cream cheese
1 chorizo sausage
¼ cup parmesan cheese, grated
½ tsp cumin
½ tsp Italian seasoning
Salt
Black pepper

Directions:

1. Set oven to 375 F.
2. Add parmesan cheese, pepper, garlic, cream cheese and eggs to a bowl and use a hand mixer to combine until smooth.
3. Coat baking pan with cooking spray and spread mixture in pan before baking for 15 minutes.
4. While crust bakes, heat a skillet and season beef with basil, salt, pepper, cumin, Italian seasoning, and turmeric. Cook for 10 minutes.
5. Remove crust from oven and cool for 10 minutes. Top crust with tomato sauce and cheese along with the meat.
6. Bake for an additional 10 minutes and broil for 5 minutes.
7. Cool, slice and serve.

(Calories 145 | Total Fats 11.3g | Net Carbs: 1.2g | Protein 8.2g)

No-Bread Cheeseburger

(Total Time: 20 MIN| **S**erve: 2)

Ingredients:

½ lb. ground beef
½ onion, chopped
1 tsp salt
1 tsp pepper
4 slices American cheddar
4 bacon strips, cooked and chopped
4 butter or romaine lettuce leaves
4 Tbsp mayonnaise

Directions:

1. Heat a cast iron skillet over medium heat. Add the ground beef and sauté with the onions. Cook until the beef is no longer pink.
2. Season the beef with the garlic powder, salt, and pepper.
3. Reduce the heat to low and then top the beef with the slices of cheese. Cover and cook for 3 minutes, or until the cheese has melted.
4. Scoop the cooked "burger patties" on the top of the lettuce leaves and dollop mayonnaise on top.
5. Serve immediately.

(Calories 224 | Total Fats 7.1g | Net Carbs: 3.2g | Protein 34.8g)

Ham and Cheese Stromboli

(Total Time: 35 MIN| **Serve:** 4)

Ingredients:

1 ¼ cups mozzarella cheese
3 Tbsp coconut flour
1 tsp Italian seasoning
3 ½ oz cheddar cheese
4 Tbsp almond flour
1 egg
4 oz ham
Salt
Black pepper

Directions:

1. Preheat oven to 400 F. Place mozzarella into a microwave safe dish and melt for 1 minute, stirring occasionally.
2. Mix flour and seasoning together in a bowl, then add melted cheese and combine thoroughly.
3. Cool for a minute before adding egg and mix together.
4. Place parchment paper on a baking sheet and place mozzarella dough onto paper, top with another paper and use a rolling pin to flatten.
5. Use a knife to slice dough diagonally from edge to middle of the dough, leaving 4 inches of dough unsliced.
6. Place ham and cheese on unsliced section of dough and cover with sliced section
7. Bake for 15-20 minutes until the top is browned. Serve warm.

(Calories 306 | Total Fats 21.8g | Net Carbs: 4.7g | Protein 25.6g)

Squash Spaghetti Lasagna Dish

(Total Time: 1 HR 30 MIN| Serve: 14)

Ingredients:

2 1/2 lbs. ground beef
2 large spaghetti squash
7 ounces whole milk ricotta cheese
7 ounces mozzarella cheese, sliced
4 cups marinara sauce
Coconut or olive oil for greasing

Directions:

1. Preheat oven to 375 F. Grease a large baking dish with coconut or olive oil.
2. Split the spaghetti squash and lay face down into a large glass dish and fill with water. Bake for 40-45 minutes.
3. While the spaghetti squash is cooking, cook the ground meat and the marinara sauce in a large saucepan. Once combined, set aside.
4. When the spaghetti squash is done, scrape the meat of the squash to form spaghetti.
5. Assemble the lasagna in a large greased pan, start with a layer of spaghetti squash, then the meat sauce, then slices of mozzarella, then ricotta, then repeat until ingredients are exhausted.
6. Bake for 30-35 minutes, until the top layer of cheese is browning. Serve hot or keep refrigerated.

(Calories 437 | Total Fats 27.7g | Net Carbs: 16.4g | Protein 28g)

Spicy Italian Sausage and Spinach Casserole

(Total Time: 1 HR 5 MIN| **Serve**: 10)

Ingredients:

16 oz. spicy Italian sausage
2 1/2 cups frozen spinach
12 eggs
8 oz. cheddar
1 onion
9 oz. cherry tomatoes
1 green pepper, chopped
12 Tbsp heavy cream
Garlic powder
Onion powder
Salt and ground pepper to taste
Coconut or olive oil

Directions:

1. Preheat oven to 350 F. Grease casserole dish with coconut or olive oil.
2. In microwave cook the spinach. Chop the spicy Italian sausage and cook in a frying pan until browned. Remove to the big bowl and set aside.
3. In the same frying pan, cook the sliced onion and pepper. Transfer to the bowl with spinach.
4. Whisk together the eggs, spices and a heavy cream. Add the cheese to the bowl and combine, then add the egg mixture and combine.
5. Transfer to a greased casserole dish and add cherry tomatoes.
6. Cook in preheated oven for 50 minutes. Serve hot.

(Calories 343 | Total Fats 25g | Net Carbs: 6.2g | Protein 22g)

Mediterranean Pecorino Romano Breaded Cutlets

(Total Time: 30 MIN| **S**erve: 3)

Ingredients:

6 pork cutlets
1/2 cup grated pecorino romano cheese
2 Tbsp fresh lemon juice
2 Tbsp water
1 Tbsp olive oil
1 Tbsp green pepper, minced
1 Tbsp garlic, minced
Salt and ground black pepper to taste

Directions:

1. Heat a greasing frying pan to medium.
2. Pour water, lemon juice, olive oil, minced pepper, and garlic into a bowl. Season with salt and pepper to taste. Mix well.
3. In a separate bowl, pour grated pecorino romano cheese.
4. Dip each cutlet first in liquid dressing and then in cheese.
5. Cook cutlets in pan for about 15-20 minutes. Serve hot.

(Calories 395 | Total Fats 38g | Net Carbs: 2.5g | Protein 9.1g)

Pumpkin Chili

(Total Time: 1 Hr 20 MIN| **Serve: 8**)

Ingredients:

2 lbs. ground beef
1 can (15 oz.) pumpkin puree
1 Tbsp pumpkin pie spice
3 cups 100% tomato juice
3 tomatoes, diced
1 red bell pepper
1 yellow onion
2 tsp cumin
1 Tbsp chili powder
2 tsp cayenne pepper
Ghee or coconut oil

Directions:

1. In a large frying pan greased with ghee or coconut oil, brown the meat over medium heat.
2. Chop the onion and pepper and add into the pot with the meat. Cook 3-5 minutes or until the onions become translucent.
3. Add in the rest of the ingredients and let simmer on Low for 30 minutes.
4. Season chili with salt and pepper to taste and cook for another 30 minutes.
5. Serve hot.

(Calories 354 | Total Fats 25g | Net Carbs: 9.8g | Protein 21g)

Monterey Jack Steak

(Total Time: 20 MIN| **Serve:** 4)

Ingredients:

1 lb. shaved steak
4 slices Monterey Jack cheese
2 Tbsp mayonnaise
1 Tbsp Dijon mustard
1/4 cup chopped green peppers
1/4 cup chopped onions
1 Tbsp minced garlic
1 Tbsp olive oil
1 Tbsp ghee

Directions:

1. In a large frying pan, add ghee and olive oil to warm over medium heat. Add onions, green peppers, and garlic. Cook until soft, about 2-3 minutes. Add shaved steak and cook until browned several minutes.
2. Turn heat down to low. Add Dijon mustard and mayonnaise and mix.
3. Add Monterey Jack cheese on top of the steak and let melt until cheese is melted throughout about 1 minute.
4. Serve hot.

(Calories 345 | Total Fats 25g | Net Carbs: 4.3g | Protein 24g)

Cheesy Keto Pizza

(Total Time: 20 MIN| **Serve:** 7)

Ingredients:

1 lb. ground beef
2 beef sausage
1 cup chopped romaine lettuce
2 Tbsp yellow onions
3 Tbsp chopped dill pickle
1 1/2 cups parmesan cheese
1/2 cup colby cheese, shredded
1 1/2 cups cheddar, shredded
1/4 Tbsp paprika
1/4 tsp Old Bay seasoning
1/4 tsp garlic powder
1/4 tsp onion powder
2 Tbsp organic Thousand Island dressing
Mustard to taste
1/4 tsp sea salt
1/4 tsp ground black pepper
Olive oil
2 Tbsp water

Directions:

1. In a frying pan greased with olive oil, add 1 cup Parmesan cheese evenly and then on top, 1 cup shredded Cheddar.
2. Leave to cook 2-3 minutes; use a spatula to lift the edges and underneath of the pizza, and slide out onto a flat surface. Allow cooling.
3. Repeat the same process, for the second pizza crust. Once done, set both cheese crusts aside.
4. Use a spatula and evenly spread Thousand Island dressing over the cheese crusts
5. In a frying pan, add ground beef and cook until browned. Add Old Bay seasoning, garlic powder, onion powder paprika, 2 Tbsp water, salt, ground black pepper to taste. Mix and set to simmer on low.

6. Finally, add in chopped hot dogs into slices and simmer for about 4-5 minutes.
7. Place chopped lettuce over your pizza crust.
8. In a bowl, place your pickles, onions, colby cheese, and set aside.
9. On top of each cheese crust, add about a cup of the ground meat and hot dog mixture and spread evenly. Sprinkle with onions and pickles.
10. Drizzle mustard on top.
11. Sprinkle with more cheese if you like and serve.

(Calories 511 | Total Fats 39g | Net Carbs: 2.7g | Protein 33g)

Sausage & Cheese Bombs

(Total Time: 25 MIN| Serve: 12)

Ingredients:

12. oz. pork sausage
¾ cup sharp cheddar cheese, shredded
12 mozzarella cheese cubes

Directions:

1. Crumble the sausage and combine with the shredded cheese in a bowl.
2. Divide into 12 patties and place 1 mozzarella cube at the center of each patty.
3. Cover the cheese with the meat and create a ball.
4. Heat your fryer up to 375 degrees and fry the meatballs until golden brown.
5. Serve with a keto-friendly marinara sauce on the side.

(Calories 173 | Total Fats 14g | Net Carbs: 1g | Protein 10g)

Spicy Spinach Casserole

(Total Time: 60 MIN| Serve: 10)

Ingredients:

2 1/2 cups spinach, drained
2 lbs. ground pork/beef
16 oz. cream cheese
10 Tbsp sour cream
8 oz. emmenthal cheese, shredded
2 cups pepper sauce
1 onion
1 red pepper
4 tsp taco seasoning
Sliced jalapeños to taste

Directions:

1. Preheat oven to 350 F. Grease one 8" square and a 9x13 baking dish.
2. Chop and sauté some jalapenos with chopped peppers and onions. Transfer to a bowl and set aside.
3. Add the spinach to the pan and cook until thawed completely. Move the spinach to the prep bowl.
4. In a frying pan, add ground pork/meat and cook until browned well. Add taco seasoning and mix. Remove from fire and set aside.
5. In a bowl, add sour cream, mozzarella, and cream cheese. Add in peppers, onion, spinach and ground meat.
6. Transfer this mixture to prepared and greased baking dish and bake for 40 minutes.
7. Serve hot or cold.

(Calories 460 | Total Fats 37g | Net Carbs: 5.3g | Protein 25g)

Bolognese Squash Spaghetti

(Total Time: 1 HR 40 MIN| **Serve:** 5)

Ingredients:

1 lb. ground beef
2 1/2 cups spaghetti squash
1 egg
3/4 cup marinara Sauce
1 cup grated parmesan cheese
1 cups shredded mozzarella cheese
1 tsp chili powder
1/2 tsp oregano
1/2 tsp parsley (fresh and chopped)
1/2 tsp basil
1 tsp crushed red pepper flakes
2 tsp of garlic minced
Sea salt and ground fresh pepper to taste
Ghee

Directions:

1. Preheat oven to 350 F.
2. Roast your spaghetti squash in the oven for about one hour.
3. In a saucepan, heat Marinara sauce; add oregano, parsley, basil and red pepper flakes. Cover and let simmer for a few minutes. Mix meatball ingredients in a bowl and roll into quarter-sized mini meatballs.
4. In a frying pan heat, the ghee and cook meatballs covered. After 3 minutes, flip when halfway browned.
5. Once the meatballs are cooked through, transfer them into the sauce.
6. In a small bread pan, layer spaghetti squash, sauce, meatballs and mozzarella.
7. Bake on 25 for 30 minutes. Serve hot.

(Calories 446 | Total Fats 30g | Net Carbs: 9.1g | Protein 32g)

Baked Pork Chops in Sweet-Sour Marinade

(Total Time: 1 HR 10 MIN| **Serve:** 10)

Ingredients:

4.4 lbs. pork chops
1 cup apple cider vinegar
1 cup erythritol
4 Tbsp soy sauce
1 cup apple cider vinegar
1 tsp ginger
1 tsp pepper
Coconut or olive oil for greasing

Directions:

1. Preheat oven to 350 F.
2. In a food processor, add all of the ingredients (except the pork chops).
3. Blend well to make the marinade.
4. In a greased pan, place all of the pork chops and pour the marinade over them.
5. Cook for 60 minutes in a preheated oven, flipping after 30 minutes.
6. Once ready, place chops on a serving plate and enjoy your lunch.

(Calories 307 | Total Fats 6g | Net Carbs: 11.43g | Protein 45g)

Grilled Cheese and Ham Sandwich

(Total Time: 30 MIN| Serve: 2)

Ingredients:

For buns:
2 eggs
1 ½ Tbsp butter, salted
1 tsp coconut flour
¾ cup almond flour
2 Tbsp coconut oil
1 tsp baking powder
¼ tsp salt

Filling:
4 deli ham slices
2 cheddar cheese slices
1 Tbsp butter, salted
2 muenster cheese slices

Directions:

1. Set oven to 350 F.
2. Place almond flour, baking powder in a bowl and mix together.
3. Put coconut oil and butter in a microwavable dish and heat until melted then add to dry mix. Combine until mixture gets doughy.
4. Beat eggs and add to dough mixture then put in coconut flour.
5. Grease cupcake molds and add batter to each about ¾ ways filled. Baked for 18 minutes and take from oven, allow to cool and slice into two horizontally.
6. Use cheese and ham to fill buns, melt butter in a skillet and place sandwiches in the pan. Cook for 3 minutes on each side until golden and cheese melts.
7. Serve.

(Calories 272 | Total Fats 24.2g | Net Carbs: 1.8g | Protein 11.3g)

Beef Sausage, Bacon & Broccoli Casserole

(Total Time: 45 MIN| Serve: 8)

Ingredients:

1.1 lbs beef sausage

1/2 head of broccoli

8 slices of bacon

½ cups cream

1 Tbsp Dijon mustard

1 cup cheddar cheese, grated

Directions:

1. Preheat oven to 350 F.
2. Slice the sausage and place in a small baking dish.
3. Slice the bacon and add to the sausage.
4. Break the broccoli into florets and arrange between the meat.
5. Mix the cream and mustard in a bowl and pour it all over the casserole, then top with the cheese.
6. Bake in the oven for 35 minutes.

(Calories 300 | Total Fats 25g | Net Carbs: 3g | Protein 20g)

Cheesy Bacon Spinach Log

(Total Time: 1 HR 15 MIN| **Serve**: 5)

Ingredients:

2 ½ cups cheddar cheese, shredded
2 Tbsp chipotle seasoning
30 bacon slices
2 tsp Mrs. Dash seasoning
5 cups spinach

Directions:

1. Set oven to 375 F.
2. Place bacon in a weaving pattern on a baking sheet lined with foil and season with spices.
3. Top bacon with cheese, leaving a 1-inch space all around the edge. Add spinach and push it down to compact before rolling the bacon together into a log.
4. Sprinkle with salt and place into oven for 60 minutes.
5. Cool for 15 minutes and slice.
6. Serve.

(Calories 432 | Total Fats 38.2g | Net Carbs: 3g | Protein 32.8g)

Savoury Mince

(Total Time: 20 MIN| Serve: 5)

Ingredients:

4 Tbsp coconut oil
2.2 lbs beef/chicken/lamb/pork/ostrich mince
2 onions finely diced
4 cups vegetables (green/red/yellow/orange peppers, mushroom, tomatoes, celery, baby marrows, and spinach) finely diced
4 carrots finely grated
1 packet gluten-free gravy
½ cup tomato paste
1 cup chicken stock

Directions:

1. Heat coconut oil in a pan and fry chopped onion,
2. Add beef mince with tomato paste and fry.
3. Add chopped vegetables and grated carrot to the cooked mince.
4. Continue to cook on a low heat, until the vegetables are well cooked.
5. If your mixture seems to be drying out, keep adding chicken stock to keep at the right consistency.
6. The longer you cook this mixture, the more the flavors will infuse through the mince.
7. Add gluten-free gravy.

(Calories 596 | Total Fats 14.3g | Net Carbs: 28g | Protein 65.5g)

Chorizo Stuffed Bell Peppers

(Total Time: 45 MIN| **Serve:** 2)

Ingredients:

3 large bell peppers, cut in half, core and seeds removed
½ lb. spicy chorizo sausage, crumbled
2 cloves of garlic
1 onion, chopped
6 organic eggs
¼ cup almond milk, unsweetened
1 cup cheddar cheese, shredded
½ Tbsp ghee
Salt and pepper to taste

Directions:

1. Set oven to 350 F.
2. Heat the ghee in a non-stick pan over medium heat and cook the chorizo crumbles. Set aside.
3. Using the same pan, add the onions and garlic and sauté for a few minutes. Turn off the heat and set aside.
4. In a bowl, stir together the eggs, milk, cheddar, and season with salt and pepper.
5. Add the chorizo into the bowl with the eggs and stir well.
6. Place the bell pepper halves in an oven-safe dish filled with a ¼ inch of water.
7. Scoop the chorizo and egg mixture into the bell peppers and place the dish into the oven to bake for 35 minutes.
8. Serve warm.

(Calories 631 | Total Fats 46g | Net Carbs: 13g | Protein 44g)

Sour Sausages with Shallots and Kalamata Olives

(Total Time: 30 MIN| Serve: 6)

Ingredients:

1 lb sausages chopped
4 shallots, finely chopped
1/2 cup lemon juice (2 lemons)
16 black and green kalamata olives
2 Tbsp whole grain mustard
4 Tbsp extra virgin olive oil
Salt and ground black pepper to taste

Directions:

1. Preheat oven to 400F. Grease a roasting pan and place in the sausages and chopped shallots.
2. Roast for 20 minutes.
3. When ready, remove the meat from the sausages and season with salt and freshly ground pepper to taste.
4. Pour the lemon juice into the roasting tin.
5. Add the mustard and chopped olives and simmer gently for 2-3 minutes. Pour lemon mixture over the sausages and shallots.
6. Place on serving plate andenjoy.

(Calories 408 | Total Fats 16.67g | Net Carbs: 6.78g | Protein 18.48g)

Sour and Spicy Goat Skewers

(Total Time: 25 MIN| **S**erve: 2)

Ingredients:

1 lb boneless goat loin, cut into cubes
2 Tbsp lime juice (freshly squeezed)
1 cup coconut yogurt
1/4 tsp ground ginger
3/4 tsp turmeric
1/2 tsp ground cumin
1 Tbsp ground coriander
1/2 tsp salt
Skewers

Directions:

1. In a medium bowl, stir together coconut yogurt, lime juice, and all seasonings; mix well.
2. Add the goat meat cubes to the bowl, stir to coat with the marinade, cover and refrigerate for 6-8 hours.
3. Remove the meat from the marinade, pat lightly with paper towels to dry.
4. Place meat evenly on the skewers. Grill over medium-hot coals, turning frequently, for about 10 minutes until nicely brown.
5. Serve and enjoy.

(Calories 342.93 | Total Fats 9.79g | Net Carbs: 7.96g | Protein 26.77g)

Meaty Bagels

(Total Time: 60 MIN| Serve: 2)

Ingredients:

3 small onions, minced

2 Tbsp organic butter

4 lbs ground pork

4 organic eggs

1 ¼ cups all-natural tomato sauce

2 tsp paprika

Salt and pepper to taste

Directions:

1. Set the oven at 400 F.
2. Melt the butter in a non-stick pan over medium heat. Add the minced onions and sauté for a few minutes, until the onions turn translucent. Set aside
3. In a large bowl, combine the ground pork, eggs, and tomato sauce. Season with salt, pepper, paprika and then add the sautéed onions.
4. Combine the ingredients, using your hands, and then form into 12 balls.
5. Flatten the middle of the ball to make it look like a bagel and then place on top of a baking sheet lined with parchment paper.
6. Bake in the oven to bake for 40 minutes, or until cooked through.

(Calories 805 | Total Fats 26.4g | Net Carbs: 9.9g | Protein 126g)

Madras Lamb Curry

(Total Time: 5 HR 20 MIN| **Serve: 8**)

Ingredients:

8 fatty lamb chops
6 Tbsp coconut milk
2 cups water
3 Tbsp red curry paste
2 Tbsp Thai fish sauce
1 Tbsp dried onion flakes
2 Tbsp dried Thai or fresh red chilies
1 Tbsp xylitol
1 Tbsp ground cumin
1 Tbsp ground coriander
1/8 tsp ground cloves
1/8 tsp ground nutmeg
1 Tbsp ground ginger

To Serve:

2 Tbsp coconut milk powder
1 Tbsp red curry paste
2 Tbsp xylitol
¼ tsp xanthan gum (optional)
1/4 cup cashews, roughly chopped
1/4 cup fresh cilantro, chopped

Directions:

1. Place the raw lamb chops in a large slow cooker.
2. Add the coconut milk, water, red curry paste, fish sauce, onion flakes, chilies, xylitol, ginger, nutmeg, cloves, coriander, and cumin. Cover with lid and cook on high for 5 hours.
3. Just before serving, remove the meat from slow cooker and place on another dish. Then stir into the sauce the 2 Tbsp coconut milk powder, 1 Tbsp curry paste, 2 Tbsp sweetener, and 1/4 tsp xanthan gum (if using).
4. Shred meat and stir into the sauce, along with cashews. Garnish with coriander before serving.

(Calories 190 | Total Fats 11g | Net Carbs: 4g | Protein 18g)

Balsamic Pork

(Total Time: 8 HR 15 MIN| **Serve:** 4)

Ingredients:

1 lb. pork roast
1/2 cup balsamic vinegar
1/3 cup honey
2 tsp fresh rosemary
1/2 tsp thyme (dried)
2 bay leaves
2 tsp salt
1/4 tsp black pepper

Directions:

1. Place pork roast in the slow cooker.
2. Mix all ingredients in a bowl and pour over roast.
3. Cook on low for 6-8 hours, or high for 4-6, depending on the size of the roast.
4. Remove the cooked roast from the slow-cooker.
5. Cover and keep warm.
6. Pour the remaining sauce from slow cooker into a saucepan and bring to the boil.
7. Let it reduce by about half.
8. Slice the roast and pour the sauce over top.

(Calories 379 | Total Fats 11.45g | Net Carbs: 32.7g | Protein 35g)

Bolognese Mince

(Total Time: 6 HR 20 MIN| **Serve:** 8)

Ingredients:

2.2 lbs beef mince
2 brown onions, diced
4 cloves garlic, crushed
1 cup tomato paste
2 Tbsp chicken stock powder or 2 Knorr Jelly Pots
1 tin tomato soup
1 tin diced tomato
1/4 cup sweet chili sauce
1 Tbsp oregano
2 bay leaves
2 cups water
1 cup finely grated carrot
3-4 finely chopped sticks of celery
2 cups finely chopped mushrooms

Directions:

1. In a frying pan, add the olive oil and heat. Brown the beef and add the onions and garlic. Cook for 2 minutes more.
2. Mix the tomato paste into the pan and cook for another 2 minutes.
3. Pour both mixtures into the slow cooker and add the rest of the ingredients and stir.
4. Cook on low for 6 hours or high for 3 hours.

(Calories 187 | Total Fats 5.2g | Net Carbs: 8g | Protein 27g)

Smoky Pork Cassoulet

(Total Time: 5 HR 15 MIN| **Serve:** 6)

Ingredients:

1 pack bacon, fried and then crumbled
2 cups chopped onion
1 tsp dried thyme
1/2 tsp dried rosemary
3 garlic cloves, crushed
1/2 tsp salt
1/2 tsp freshly ground black pepper
2 cans diced tomatoes, drained
1.1 lbs boneless pork loin roast, trimmed and cut into 2cm cubes
1.2 lbs smoked sausage, cut into 1cm cubes
8 tsp finely shredded fresh parmesan cheese
8 tsp chopped fresh flat-leaf parsley

Directions:

1. Fry bacon onion, thyme, rosemary, and garlic, then add salt, pepper, and tomatoes; bring to a boil.
2. Remove from heat.
3. Place all ingredients in the slow cooker, alternating the meat with the tomato sauce until finished. Cover and cook on low for 5 hours. Sprinkle with parmesan cheese and parsley when cooked

(Calories 258 | Total Fats 12.6g | Net Carbs: 10.8g | Protein 27g)

Tomato Bredie

(Total Time: 4 HR 20 MIN| Serve: 8)

Ingredients:

1 Tbsp olive oil

3.3 lbs or mutton chops or 1.5kgs of stewing lamb

2 Tbsp almond flour, psyllium husk or finely ground chia seeds

1 large onion, chopped

3.3 lbs fresh tomatoes, finely chopped

1 tsp salt

1/2 tsp freshly ground black pepper

2 bay leaves

1 tsp xylitol

1 Tbsp white vinegar

1 dash Worcestershire sauce

1 cube beef or lamb stock

Directions:

1. Heat oil over medium-high heat in a large, heavy-bottomed saucepan.
2. Dredge meat in almond flour or ground chia seeds and cook in hot oil until well browned.
3. Stir in onions, and cook for about 5 minutes or until soft. Mix in tomatoes.
4. Season with salt, black pepper, white peppercorns, bay leaves, xylitol, vinegar, Worcestershire sauce, and beef bouillon cube.
5. Cover, reduce heat and simmer for 3-4 hours on low.

(Calories 385 | Total Fats 15g | Net Carbs: 9g | Protein 50g)

Chapter 8 Soups & Stews

Lemon Chicken Stew

(Total Time: 6 HR 30 MIN| **Serve:** 10)

Ingredients:

2 carrots, chopped
2 ribs celery, chopped
1 onion, chopped
20 large green olives
4 cloves garlic, crushed
2 bay leaves
½ tsp dried oregano
¼ tsp salt
¼ tsp pepper
12 boneless skinless chicken thighs
¾ cup chicken stock
¼ cup almond flour or psyllium husk or finely ground
Chia seeds
2 Tbsp lemon juice
½ cup chopped fresh parsley
Grated zest of 1 lemon

Directions:

1. In slow cooker, combine carrots, celery, onion, olives, garlic, bay leaves, oregano, salt, and pepper.
2. Arrange chicken pieces on top of vegetables. Add broth and ¾ cup water. Cover and cook on low for 5-1/2 to 6 hours or until juices run clear when chicken is pierced. Discard bay leaves.
3. Whisk flour with 1 cup of the cooking liquid until smooth; whisk in lemon juice. Pour mixture into slow cooker; cook, covered, on high until thickened, about 15 minutes.
4. Mix parsley with lemon zest; serve sprinkled over chicken mixture. Enjoy!

(Calories 331 | Total Fats 15.7g | Net Carbs: 3.9g | Protein 40.5g)

Beef Chuck Cabbage Stew

(Total Time: 9 HR 15 MIN| Serve: 6)

Ingredients:

1 packet frozen baby carrots
2 medium onions, roughly chopped
1 small cabbage cored, and cut into 8 wedges
8 garlic cloves, peeled and smashed
2 bay leaves
8 pieces of beef chuck with marrow
Salt and freshly ground pepper to taste
2 tins diced tomatoes, drained
1 cup chicken stock
Side salad to serve

Directions:

1. Place the baby carrots and chopped onions into the bottom of the slow cooker.
2. Layer the cabbage wedges on top.
3. Add crushed garlic cloves and bay leaves
4. Season the beef shanks with salt and pepper (by the way, feel free to be pretty heavy-handed with the S&P).
5. Add beef shanks on top of vegetables.
6. Pour in the diced tomatoes and broth before putting on the lid.
7. Set the slow cooker on low for 9 hours.
8. Serve with salad on the side.

(Calories 234 | Total Fats 16g | Net Carbs: 5g | Protein 16g)

Hearty Beef Stew

(Total Time: 8 HR 20 MIN| **Serve:** 6)

Ingredients:

2.2 lbs stewing beef

3 Tbsp olive oil

2 cups beef stock

1 packet streaky bacon – cooked crisp and crumbled

2 cans diced tomatoes – juice drained

2 cups mixed bell peppers – chopped

2 cups mushrooms – quartered

2 ribs celery – chopped

1 large carrot – chopped

1 small onion – chopped

4 large cloves garlic – minced

2 Tbsp organic tomato paste

2 Tbsp Worcestershire sauce

2 tsp sea salt

1 ½ tsp black pepper

1 tsp garlic powder

1 tsp onion powder

1 tsp dried oregano

Directions:

1. Set slow cooker on low.
2. In a large pan over medium heat, sear the beef in olive oil, browning on both sides. Transfer to slow cooker.
3. Pour beef stock, bacon, tomatoes, bell peppers, mushrooms, celery, carrot, onion, garlic, tomato paste, Worcestershire sauce, sea salt, black pepper, garlic powder, onion powder, and dried oregano into the slow cooker.
4. Cover and cook on low 6-8 hours.
5. Serve in bowls for a hearty keto feast.

(Calories 280 | Total Fats 6g | Net Carbs: 20g | Protein 18g)

Curried Chicken Stew

(Total Time: 8 HR 20 MIN| Serve: 8)

Ingredients:

8 bone-in chicken thighs
2 Tbsp olive oil or coconut oil
6 carrots cut into 2-inch pieces
1 sweet onion cut into thin wedges
1 cup unsweetened coconut milk
1/4 cup milk (or hot) curry paste
Toasted almonds, coriander, and fresh green or red chili

Directions:

1. Cook chicken in a pan skin side down, in hot olive oil for 8 minutes, or until browned.
2. Remove from heat; drain and discard fat.
3. In a slow cooker, combine carrots and onion.
4. Whisk together half the coconut milk and the curry paste, pour over carrots and onion
5. Place chicken, skin side up on top of vegetables and pour over olive oil from pan.
6. Cover and cook on high for 3.5 to 4 hours, or on low for 7 to 8 hours.
7. Remove chicken from slow cooker. Skim excess fat from sauce in the cooker, and then stir in remaining coconut milk.
8. Serve stew in bowls. Top each serving with toasted almonds, coriander, fresh chili and a dollop of yogurt or crème Fraiche.

(Calories 321 | Total Fats 22g | Net Carbs: 20g | Protein 14g)

Curried Cauliflower & Chicken Stew

(Total Time: 6 HR 20 MIN| **Serve:** 8)

Ingredients:

3½ Tbsp coconut oil
1 bunch fresh mint or coriander leaves, chopped
1 head cauliflower, broken into large florets
Freshly ground black pepper
1½ tsp salt
6 bone-in skinless chicken thighs, about 1.1kg
2 cups whole milk plain yogurt
3 cups chicken stock, low-sodium canned
1/2 cup prepared red curry paste (depending on heat required)
5-cm piece fresh ginger, minced
6 cloves garlic, minced
1 lemon cut in wedges

Directions:

1. Heat the oil; add the garlic and ginger and cook. Add the curry paste and continue to cook. Whisk the broth in the pan; then pour the liquid into a slow cooker. Whisk the yogurt into the liquid.
2. Season the chicken all over with salt and pepper.
3. Add the chicken and remaining salt to the slow cooker. Cover and cook on high for 6 hours, adding cauliflower about halfway through cooking.
4. Scatter freshly torn mint or coriander on top. Serve with a wedge of lemon.

(Calories 343 | Total Fats 15g | Net Carbs: 31g | Protein 23g)

Farmhouse Lamb & Cabbage Stew

(Total Time: 6 HR 50 MIN| Serve: 8)

Ingredients:

2 Tbsp olive oil or coconut oil
1.1 lb lamb chops, bone in
1 lamb or beef stock cube
2 cups water
1 cabbage, finely chopped
1 onion, sliced
2 carrots, chopped
2 sticks celery, chopped
1 tsp dried thyme
1 Tbsp balsamic vinegar
1 Tbsp almond flour or psyllium husk

Directions:

1. Set the slow cooker to low.
2. Heat oil in a large frying pan and brown the lamb chops.
3. Add lamb to the slow cooker with remaining ingredients, mix until ingredients are evenly distributed.
4. Cook on low for 6- to hours. Then remove bones from lamb.
5. For thicker a sauce, 30 minutes before serving ladle ¼ cup of the sauce into a small bowl and whisk almond flour/psyllium husk into it with a fork. Return mixture to the slow cooker bowl, stir through and leave for a further 30minutes.

(Calories 180 | Total Fats 4g | Net Carbs: 9g | Protein 26g)

Seafood Stew

(Total Time: 6 HR 50 MIN| Serve: 8)

Ingredients:

1 Tbsp olive oil

2 onions, diced

4 stalks celery, chopped

4 garlic cloves, minced

1 tsp dried oregano

½ tsp ground black pepper

1 tTsp tomato paste

1 Tbsp flour

3 cups chicken stock

1 can tomato, onion and chili mix

1 -2 cup tomato cocktail juice

4 chicken breasts cut into bite-size pieces

2 packets mixed frozen seafood (you can add extra mussels in at the end)

2 peppers (red and green)

1 jalapeno pepper, chopped

¼cup parsley, chopped

1 tsp chili powder

1 pinch cayenne pepper

1 Tbsp butter

Directions:

1. In a large pan, heat the olive oil and fry onions and celery
2. Add garlic, oregano, peppercorns. Stir in tomato paste and almond flour and cook another minute.
3. Add chicken stock, tomatoes and tomato juice and bring to a boil. Continue to cook for about 3-5 more minutes. Remove from heat and transfer mixture to slow cooker.
4. Add chicken and stir to combine. Cover and cook on high for 3 hours, or low for 6 hours.
5. Stir in mixed bags of frozen seafood and parsley. Cover and cook on high for 30 minutes.
6. Add extra mussels just before serving, if desired.

(Calories 177 | Total Fats 4g | Net Carbs: 15g | Protein 21g)

Rosemary Garlic Beef Stew

(Total Time: 4 HR 20 MIN| Serve: 8)

Ingredients:

4 medium carrots, sliced

4 sticks celery, sliced

1 medium onion, diced

2 tbsp olive oil

4 garlic cloves, minced

1.5 lbs beef stewing meat (shin or chuck)

Salt and pepper

¼ cup almond flour

2 cups beef stock

2 Tbsp Dijon mustard

1 Tbsp Worcestershire sauce

1 Tbsp soy sauce

1 Tbsp xylitol

½ Tbsp dried rosemary

½ tsp thyme

Directions:

1. Add onion, carrots, and celery into a slow cooker.
2. Add stewing meat in a large bowl and season with pepper and salt.
3. Add the almond flour and toss the meat until well coated.
4. Fry the garlic in the hot oil for about one minute.
5. Add the seasoned meat and all the flour from the bottom of the bowl to the pan.
6. Cook the meat without stirring for a few minutes to allow it to brown on one side.
7. Flip and repeat until all the sides of the beef are browned.
8. Add the browned beef to the slow cooker and stir to combine with the vegetables.
9. Add the beef stock, Dijon mustard, Worcestershire sauce, soy sauce, xylitol, thyme, and rosemary to the skillet.
10. Stir to combine all ingredients and dissolve the browned bits from the bottom of the skillet.
11. Once everything is dissolved, then pour the sauce over the ingredients in the slow cooker.

12. Cover slow cooker with lid and cook on high for four hours.
13. After cooking, remove the lid and stir stew well and, using a fork, shred the beef into pieces.
14. Taste the stew and adjust the seasoning.

(Calories 275 | Total Fats 10g | Net Carbs: 24g | Protein 22g)

Creamy Chicken & Pumpkin Stew

(Total Time: 5 HR| Serve: 6)

Ingredients:

1.3 lb chicken boneless chicken breast
1 1/4 cups chicken stock
1 can evaporate milk (full cream)
1/3 cup of sour cream or crème Fraiche
1 Tbsp minced garlic
½ cup grated mature cheddar cheese
Fresh or frozen finely chopped pumpkin
Salt and pepper to taste

Directions:

1. In a crock pot, combine all ingredients.
2. Cover and turn crock pot on low. Cook for 4.5 hours on low, or until both chicken and pumpkin are cooked and soft.
3. Stir sauce in crock pot prior to serving.

(Calories 321 | Total Fats 12g | Net Carbs: 17g | Protein 35g)

The Best Beef Stew

(Total Time: 6 HR 50 MIN| Serve: 8)

Ingredients:

2.2 lbs beef stewing meat, (cut into bite-sized pieces)

1 tsp Salt

1 tsp pepper

1 medium onion, finely chopped

2 celery ribs, sliced

2-3 cloves of garlic, minced

1 canned tomato paste

1-liter beef stock

2 Tbsp Worcestershire sauce

2 cups frozen vegetables

1/4 cup almond flour

1/4 cup water

Directions:

1. Combine beef, celery, carrots, red onion, potatoes, salt, pepper, garlic, parsley, oregano, Worcestershire sauce, beef broth, and tomato paste in the crock pot.
2. Cook on low for 10 hours or on High for 6-7 hours.
3. Just 30 minutes before serving, combine together flour and water in small bowl and pour into the crockpot.
4. Stir until well combined.
5. Add frozen vegetables and continue cooking covered for 30 minutes.

(Calories 173 | Total Fats 4g | Net Carbs: 20g | Protein 17g)

Thai Nut Chicken

(Total Time: 5 HR 15 MIN| **Serve: 8**)

Ingredients:

8 boneless skinless chicken thighs (about 2 pounds)
½ cup coconut flour
3/4 cup creamy nut butter
1/2 cup orange juice
1/4 cup diabetic apricot jam
2 Tbsp sesame oil
2 Tbsp soy sauce
2 Tbsp teriyaki sauce
2 Tbsp hoisin sauce
1 can coconut milk
3/4 cup water
1 cup chopped roasted almonds, or any of the other nuts on green list

Directions:

1. Place coconut flour in a large re-sealable plastic bag.
2. Add chicken, a few pieces at a time, and shake to coat.
3. Transfer to a greased slow cooker.
4. In a small bowl, combine the nut butter, orange juice, jam, oil, soy sauce, teriyaki sauce, hoisin sauce and 3/4 cup coconut milk; pour over chicken. Cover and cook on low for 4-5 hours or until chicken is tender.
5. Sprinkle with nuts before serving

(Calories 363 | Total Fats 18.15g | Net Carbs: 11.6g | Protein 38.7g)

Bouillabaisse Fish Stew

(Total Time: 6 HR 55 MIN| Serve: 6)

Ingredients:

1 cup dry white wine
Juice and zest of 1 orange
2 Tbsp olive oil
1 large onion, diced
2 cloves garlic, minced
1 tsp dried basil
1/2 tsp dried thyme
1/2 tsp salt
1/4 tsp ground black pepper
4 cups fish stock; chicken stock can also be used
1 can diced tomatoes, drained
1 bay leaf
0.9 lb boneless, skinless white fish fillet (excluding cod)
0.9 lb prawns peeled and deveined
0.9 lb mussels in their shells
Juice of 1/2 lemon
1/4 cup fresh Italian (flat-leaf) parsley

Directions:

1. Heat the oil in a large pan.
2. Add the onion and fry all the vegetables until almost tender.
3. Add the garlic, basil, thyme, salt, and pepper.
4. Pour the wine and bring to a boil. Add the fish stock, orange zest, tomatoes, and bay leaf and stir to combine.
5. Pour everything into a slow cooker, cover the cooker, and cook on low for 4 to 6 hours.
6. About 30 minutes before serving, turn the cooker to high. Toss the fish and prawns with the lemon juice.
7. Stir into the broth in the cooker, cover, and cook until the fish cooks through about 20 minutes.

8. Add mussel's right at the end and allow to steam for 20 minutes with the lid on, before serving in individual bowls.

(Calories 310 | Total Fats 30g | Net Carbs: 4g | Protein 3g)

Spanish Chorizo Soup

(Total Time: 12 HR 10 MIN| Serve: 6)

Ingredients:

2 cups sweet potatoes, cubed and peeled
4 cups cabbage and carrot coleslaw mix
1 large onion, chopped
1 tsp caraway seeds
1.1 lbs chorizo halved lengthwise and cut into thick slices
4 cups chicken stock

Directions:

1. Place potatoes, coleslaw mixture, onion, caraway seeds and sausage in slow cooker. Pour stock into a pot.
2. Cover; cook on low for 10 - 12 hours or high for 5 - 6 hours.
3. You can also use beef, chicken, or pork sausages in placeof the chorizo.

(Calories 329 | Total Fats 12.4g | Net Carbs: 12g | Protein 40g)

Beef & Broccoli Stew

(Total Time: 2 HR 20 MIN| Serve: 8)

Ingredients:

1 cup beef stock
1/4 cup soy sauce
1/4 cup oyster sauce
1/4 cup xylitol
1 Tbsp sesame oil
3 cloves garlic, minced
2.2 lbs boneless beef chuck roast and thinly sliced
2 Tbsp almond flour or psyllium husk
2 heads broccoli, cut into florets

Directions:

1. In a medium bowl, whisk together beef stock, soy sauce, oyster sauce, sugar, sesame oil, and garlic.
2. Place beef into a slow cooker. Add sauce mixture and gently toss to combine. Cover and cook on low heat for 90 minutes.
3. In a small bowl, whisk together 1/4 cup water and almond flour.
4. Stir almond flour mixture and broccoli into the slow cooker. Cover and cook on high heat for an additional 30 minutes.
5. Uncover and serve.

(Calories 370 | Total Fats 18g | Net Carbs: 4g | Protein 47g)

Mussel Stew

(Total Time: 5 HR 45 MIN| **Serve:** 8)

Ingredients:

2.2 lbs fresh or frozen, cleaned mussels
3 Tbsp olive oil
4 cloves garlic, minced
1 large onion, finely diced
1 punnet mushrooms, diced
2 cans diced tomatoes
2 Tbsp oregano
½ Tbsp basil
½ tsp black pepper
1 tsp paprika
Dash red chili flakes
3/4 cup water

Directions:

1. Fry onions, garlic, shallots and mushrooms, scrape entire contents of the pan into your crockpot.
2. Add all remaining ingredients to your slow cooker, except your mussels. Cook on low for 4-5 hours, or on high for 2-3 hours. You're cooking until your mushrooms are fork tender and until the flavors meld together.
3. Once your mushrooms are cooked and your sauce is done, crank the crockpot up to high. Add cleaned mussels to the pot and secure lid tightly. Cook for 30 more minutes.
4. Ladle your mussels into bowls with plenty of broth. If any mussels didn't open up during cooking, discard.

(Calories 228 | Total Fats 9g | Net Carbs: 32g | Protein 4g)

Sweet Potato Stew

(Total Time: 6 HR 20 MIN| Serve: 6)

Ingredients:

2 cups cubed sweet potatoes

4 boneless chicken breasts

4 boneless chicken thighs

2 cups chicken stock

1 ½ cups chopped green sweet peppers

1 ¼ cup diced fresh tomatoes

¾ cup can tomatoes, onion and chili mix

1 Tbsp cajun or curry seasoning

2 cloves garlic, minced

¼ cup creamy nut butter

Fresh coriander

Chopped, roasted nuts

Directions:

1. In a slow cooker, place sweet potatoes, chicken, broth, peppers, diced tomatoes, tomatoes and green chilies mixture, cajun seasoning, and garlic.
2. Cover and cook on low-heat setting for 10 to 12 hours, or on high-heat setting for 5 to 6 hours.
3. Remove 1 cup hot liquid from cooker. Whisk the liquid with nut butter in a bowl. Add mixture to cooker.
4. Serve topped with cilantro and, if desired, peanuts.

(Calories 399 | Total Fats 21g | Net Carbs: 13.5g | Protein 37g)

Oxtail Stew

(Total Time: 9 HR 15 MIN| **Serve:** 10)

Ingredients:

3.3 lbs of oxtail
1 large pack grated cabbage
1 large pack grated carrots
2 large onions
1 large bunch of celery
1 tin of tomatoes
2 jelly stock cubes
5 pints of water
1 Tbsp crushed garlic
1 branch rosemary
2 bay leaves
½ cup cheddar cheese (optional)

Directions:

1. Place all ingredients into a slow cooker and cook on medium for 9 hours.
2. Season with salt and pepper
3. Grate ½ cup cheddar cheese on top to finish (optional).

(Calories 152 | Total Fats 7g | Net Carbs: 5.4g | Protein 16.7g)

Italian Gnocchi Soup

(Total Time: 40 MIN| Serve: 6)

Ingredients:

1.1 lbs ground spicy Italian sausage
1 small onion, diced
2 cloves garlic, minced
4 cups chicken stock or bone broth
1 red medium pepper, diced
1 cup chopped fresh or frozen spinach
½ cup heavy cream
Sea salt and freshly cracked black pepper
Optional garnish: Parmesan cheese, chopped parsley & crumbled bacon

Directions:

1. Fry sausage, onion, and garlic. Cook until the sausage is completely browned. Stirring occasionally and break up the sausage with a spoon.
2. Add in the bone broth or chicken stock and diced red peppers to the pot and bring the mixture to a simmer.
3. Reduce heat to medium-low and add the spinach and cook for an additional 5 minutes
4. Add gnocchi & cream and stir to combine.
5. Season to taste with salt and pepper.

(Calories 336 | Total Fats 17g | Net Carbs: 4.65g | Protein 40g)

Loaded Cauliflower Soup

(Total Time: 5 HR 15 MIN| Serve: 6)

Ingredients:

3 cups cauliflower, chopped
1½ cups chicken stock
1½ cups water
¼ cup milk
¼ tsp salt
1 Tbsp butter
3 cloves garlic, minced
3 Tbsp parmesan
1 cup chopped onion
8-10 spring onions
Salt to taste
¼ tsp pepper
1 Tbsp olive oil
½ tsp parsley

To Serve (optional):
1 Packet of streaky bacon, chopped, fried crisp and crumbled
1/2 cup shredded cheddar cheese
2 Tbsp sour cream

Directions:

1. Chop cauliflower into chunks, add all ingredients to a slow cooker and cover and cook on low for 5 hours.
2. Ladle into bowls. Sprinkle with Parmesan cheese and parsley. (Optional: additional bacon, shredded cheese, and sour cream for topping)

(Calories 245 | Total Fats 14.3g | Net Carbs: 21g | Protein 11.7g)

French Onion Soup

(Total Time: 8 HR 40 MIN| **Serve:** 8)

Ingredients:

1/4 cup unsalted butter

6 thyme sprigs

1 bay leaf

5 pounds large sweet onions, vertically sliced (about 16 cups)

1 Tbsp sugar

6 cups low-sodium beef stock

2 Tbsp red wine vinegar

1 1/2 tsp kosher salt

1 tsp black pepper

5 ounces gruyere cheese, shredded (about 1 1/4 cups)

Directions:

1. Place butter, thyme, and bay leaf in the bottom of a 6-quart slow cooker. Add onions; sprinkle with sugar. Cover and cook on high for 8 hours.
2. Discard thyme and bay leaf.
3. Add wine vinegar, stock, pepper and salt and stir well.
4. Cover and cook, on HIGH for 30 minutes.
5. Ladle into bowls and sprinkle gruyere cheese on top before serving.

(Calories 258 | Total Fats 12.6g | Net Carbs: 10.8g | Protein 27g)

Thai Chicken Soup

(Total Time: 4 HR 15 MIN| Serve: 8)

Ingredients:

2 Tbsp red curry paste
2 cans of coconut milk
2 cups chicken stock
2 Tbsp fish sauce
2 Tbsp xylitol
2 Tbsp nut butter
6-8 chicken breasts cut into pieces
1 red bell pepper, seeded and sliced
1 onion, thinly sliced
4-6 large grated carrots
1 heaped Tbsp fresh ginger, minced
1 Tbsp lime juice
Coriander for garnish

Directions:

1. Mix the curry paste, coconut milk, chicken stock, fish sauce, xylitol and nut butter in a slow-cooker bowl.
2. Place the chicken breast, red bell pepper, onion, grated carrots and ginger in the slow cooker, cover and cook on high for 4 hours.
3. Add in the mange tout at the end of the cooking time and cook for a ½ hour longer. Stir in lime juice and serve in bowls with coriander.

(Calories 258 | Total Fats 12.6g | Net Carbs: 10.8g | Protein 27g)

Curried Cauliflower Soup

(Total Time: 25 MIN| **Serve**: 6)

Ingredients:

1 Tbsp olive oil
1 medium spring onion
1 cup cauliflower, steamed
1 cup beef stock
1/2 cup coconut milk
10 cashew nuts
½ tsp coriander
½ tsp turmeric
½ tsp cumin
2 Tbsp fresh parsley, finely chopped
salt and pepper, to taste

Directions:

1. Place the cauliflower and onion in a large pot and add chicken stock. Stir in coriander, turmeric, cumin and a pinch of salt. Bring to a boil and let boil for 5 minutes.
2. Remove from heat. Using a hand blender, puree ingredients in the pot until smooth. Stir in the coconut milk. Serve with roasted cashew nuts and top with parsley.

(Calories 258 | Total Fats 12.6g | Net Carbs: 10.8g | Protein 27g)

Easy Everyday Chicken Soup

(Total Time: 5 HR| **Serve:** 8)

Ingredients:

3 skinned, bone-in chicken breasts
6 skinned and boned chicken thighs
1 tsp salt
1/2 tsp freshly ground pepper
1/2 tsp chicken spice seasoning
3-4 carrots sliced
4 celery ribs, sliced
1 sweet onion, chopped
2 cans evaporated milk
2 cups chicken stock

Directions:

1. Prepare Chicken: Rub chicken pieces with salt, pepper, and chicken spice seasoning. Place breasts in a slow cooker, top with thighs.
2. Add carrots and next 3 ingredients. Whisk evaporated milk and stock until smooth. Pour soup mixture over vegetables.
3. Cover with lid and cook on high 3 and half hours.
4.   Remove chicken from slow cooker and allow to cool for 10 minutes.
5. Using fork shred the chicken.
6. Stir shredded chicken into the soup-and-vegetable mixture.
7. Cover again with lid and cook on High for 1 hour.

(Calories 282 | Total Fats 18g | Net Carbs: 5.6g | Protein 24g)

Creamy Chicken & Tomato Soup

(Total Time: 9 HR 10 MIN| Serve: 8)

Ingredients:

8 frozen skinless boneless chicken breast

2 Tbsp Italian seasoning

1 Tbsp dried basil

2 cloves garlic, minced

1 large onion, chopped

2 can of coconut milk (full fat), shake before opening to avoid separation

2 cans diced tomatoes and juice

2 ¼ cups of chicken stock

1 small can of tomato paste

Sea salt and pepper to taste

Directions:

1. Put all the above ingredients into the slow cooker, cook for 9 hours on low.
2. After 9 hours take two forks and shred the chicken, set the slow cooker on warm till ready to serve.

(Calories 227 | Total Fats 3.8g | Net Carbs: 6.37g | Protein 30g)

Tomato & Basil Soup

(Total Time: 7 HR 45 MIN| **Serve:** 6)

Ingredients:

2 cans diced tomatoes, with juice
1 cup finely diced celery
1 cup finely diced carrots
1 cup finely diced onions
1 tsp dried oregano or 1 Tbsp fresh oregano
1 Tbsp dried basil or 1/4 cup fresh basil
4 cups chicken stock
½ tsp bay leaf
1 cup parmesan cheese
½ cup butter
2 cups full cream milk
1 tsp salt
¼ tsp black pepper
¼ cup almond flour or ground chia seeds

Directions:

1. Add tomatoes, celery, carrots, chicken stock, onions, oregano, basil, and bay leaf to a large slow cooker.
2. Cover and cook on low for 5-7 hours, until flavors are blended and vegetables are tender.
3. About 30 minutes before serving, melt butter over low heat and add almond flour. Stir constantly with a whisk for 5-7 minutes.
4. Slowly stir in 1 cup hot soup. Add another 3 cups and stir until smooth. Add all back into the slow cooker.
5. Stir and add the parmesan cheese, milk, salt, and pepper.
6. Cover and cook on Low for another 30 minutes or so, until ready to serve.

(Calories 269 | Total Fats 11g | Net Carbs: 4.86g | Protein 35.71g)

Beef & Cabbage Soup

(Total Time: 8 HR 15 MIN| Serve: 8)

Ingredients:

2 Tbsp olive or coconut oil

1.1 lbs ground beef mince

1/2 large onion, chopped

5 cups chopped cabbage

2 cups water

2 tins tomato puree

4 beef stock cubes

1 1/2 tsp ground cumin

1 tsp salt

1 tsp pepper

Directions:

1. Heat oil in a large pot.
2. Add ground beef and onion, and cook until beef is brown and crumbled.
3. Transfer mince with fat to a slow cooker. Add cabbage, water, tomato sauce, bouillon, cumin, salt, and pepper. Stir to dissolve stock cubes and cover.
4. Cook on high setting for 4 hours, or on low setting for 6 to 8 hours. Stir occasionally.
5. Uncover and serve.

(Calories 165 | Total Fats 8g | Net Carbs: 13.7g | Protein 11.54g)

3 Ingredients Vegetable Beef Soup

(Total Time: 8 HR 45 MIN| Serve: 4)

Ingredients:

1.1 lbs ground beef mince
2 cups tomato-vegetable juice cocktail
2 packages frozen mixed vegetables

Directions:

1. Place ground beef mince in a slow cooker. Cook over medium-high heat until evenly brown and crumbled.
2. Add juice cocktail and mixed vegetables.
3. In a slow cooker oven, simmer for 30 minutes.
4. In a slow cooker, cook 1 hour on High.
5. Then reduce heat to Low and simmer 6 to 8 hours.

(Calories 251 | Total Fats 12g | Net Carbs: 13.5g | Protein 21.3g)

Clam Chowder

(Total Time: 11 HR 15 MIN| Serve: 8)

Ingredients:

2 can minced clams in brine
4 slices bacon, cut into small pieces
3 sweet potatoes, peeled and cubed
1 cup chopped onion
1 carrot, grated
1 punnet mushrooms fried in butter and blended finely with a hand blender
1/4 tsp ground black pepper
2 cans evaporated milk

Directions:

1. In a small bowl, drain the clams and reserve the juice.
2. Add water to the juice as needed to total 1 3/4 cups liquid. Cover the clams and put in refrigerator for later.
3. In a slow cooker, combine the bacon, sweet potatoes, onion, carrot, mushrooms, ground black pepper, evaporated milk and reserved clam juice with water.
4. Cover and cook on low setting for 9 to 11 hours, or on high setting for 4 to 5 hours. Add the clams and cook on high setting for another hour.
5. Ladle into bowls and serve.

(Calories 206 | Total Fats 9.56g | Net Carbs: 21.42g | Protein 9.24g)

Mushroom Soup

(Total Time: 6 HR 55 MIN| Serve: 8)

Ingredients:

2 punnets white button mushrooms, cleaned, trimmed, and quartered

1 medium onion, roughly chopped

4 cloves garlic, sliced

7 sprigs thyme, divided

2 small lemons, halved

2 Tbsp olive oil

1 1/2 Tbsp red wine vinegar

Salt and freshly ground black pepper

1/2 cup dry sherry

2 cups milk

1 cup heavy cream

1/2 cup sour cream

3 cups chicken stock or vegetable stock

Directions:

1. Preheat oven to 375 F.
2. Place mushrooms, onions, garlic, and 5 thyme sprigs in a large bowl. Squeeze lemons into the bowl and add the squeezed lemon halves. Add vinegar and olive oil.
3. Season with salt and pepper and toss to coat.
4. Transfer to a foil-lined, rimmed baking sheet and spread into an even layer.
5. Roast in preheated oven until mushrooms release liquid, about 15 minutes.
6. Carefully drain liquid into a separate container and reserve.
7. Return mushrooms to oven and continue roasting until browned, about 30 minutes.
8. Discard lemons and thyme sprigs.
9. Transfer mushroom mixture along with drained liquid to the slow cooker.
10. Add milk, heavy cream, sour cream, sherry, and stock, along with remaining thyme sprigs.
11. Stir well and cook on low for 6 hours.
12. Discard thyme sprigs. Transfer soup to a blender and blend until you get desired consistency.
13. Serve in bowls or mugs.

(Calories 198 | Total Fats 13.2g | Net Carbs: 15.8g | Protein 5g)

Seafood Soup

(Total Time: 4 HR 15 MIN| **Serve: 8**)

Ingredients:

12 slices bacon, chopped

2 cloves garlic, minced

6 cups chicken stock

3 stalks celery, diced

2 large carrots, diced

Ground black pepper to taste

1/2 tsp red pepper flakes, or to taste

2 cups onions

2 cup uncooked prawns, peeled and deveined

1.1 lbs white fish fillets like Hake or Kingklip, cut into bite-size pieces

1 can evaporated milk

Directions:

1. Fry bacon in coconut oil or olive oil, add onion and garlic. Transfer mixture to a slow cooker.
2. Pour chicken stock into slow cooker. Add celery, and carrots into the stock. Season with black pepper and red pepper flakes.
3. Set the cooker to high, cover, and cook for 3 hours.
4. Stir prawns and fish into the soup and cook 1 more hour. Stir evaporated milk into chowder, heat thoroughly, and serve.

(Calories 281 | Total Fats 9.5g | Net Carbs: 7.8g | Protein 39g)

Cream of Broccoli & Mushroom Soup

(Total Time: 4 HR 15 MIN| Serve: 6)

Ingredients:

1 Tbsp oil

1 onion, chopped

2 packets frozen chopped broccoli, thawed

2 cans cream of celery soup

2 punnets of mushrooms fried in butter and blitzed smooth with a hand blender

1 cup shredded cheddar cheese

2 cans evaporated milk

Directions:

1. Fry the onion in coconut oil and transfer to the slow cooker.
2. Transfer the drained onion to a slow cooker.
3. Place the broccoli, cream of celery soup, mushrooms, cheddar cheese, and milk into the slow cooker.
4. Cook on low for 3-4 hours or until the broccoli is tender.
5. Serve in bowls.

(Calories 212 | Total Fats 4.7g | Net Carbs: 36.6g | Protein 10g)

Beef & Vegetable Soup

(Total Time: 8 HR 15 MIN| Serve: 8)

Ingredients:

2.2 lbs beef chuck or neck

1 can diced tomatoes, undrained

2 medium sweet potatoes, peeled and cubed

2 medium onions, diced

3 celery ribs, sliced

2 carrots, sliced

2 cups pumpkin

3 beef stock cubes

1/2 tsp salt

1/2 tsp dried basil

1/2 tsp dried oregano

1/4 tsp pepper

3 cups water

Directions:

1. Chop vegetables as indicated.
2. In a slow cooker, combine all the ingredients. Cover and cook on high for 6-8 hours.
3. Uncover, adjust seasoning and serve.

(Calories 253 | Total Fats 14.5g | Net Carbs: 10g | Protein 23g)

Cream of Carrot Soup

(Total Time: 8 HR 25 MIN| Serve: 6)

Ingredients:

1 onion, diced
2 stalks celery, diced
1 large sweet potato, diced
8 whole carrots, sliced
4 cups chicken broth stock
1 whole bay leaf
Salt and pepper, to taste
4 dashes Tabasco (or other hot sauce)
1 cup heavy cream
1 tsp parsley

Directions:

1. Add all ingredients, except parsley and heavy cream, to a slow cooker.
2. Cover and cook on low for 6-8 hours.
3. Discard bay leaf.
4. Using a hand blender, puree the vegetables.
5. Turn heat to high and stir in parsley and heavy cream.
6. Cook for another 15 minutes to allow the heavy cream to heat thoroughly.

(Calories 356 | Total Fats 31.7g | Net Carbs: 14.7g | Protein 5g)

Cream of Tomato Soup

(Total Time: 6 HR 15 MIN| Serve: 6)

Ingredients:

2 Tbsp unsalted butter
2 large onion, finely chopped
2 cans diced tomatoes with juice
1 cup chicken stock
1 cup heavy cream, warmed
1/4 tsp cayenne pepper
Salt and pepper to taste

Directions:

1. Melt butter and fry the onion. Transfer to slow cooker.
2. Add tomatoes with juice, half cup water, and stock into the cooker and stir well.
3. Cover with lid and cook on low for 5 to 6 hours.
4. Puree the soup with a blender, then stir in cream.
5. Season with pepper and salt.
6. Serve and enjoy.

(Calories 229 | Total Fats 11.5g | Net Carbs: 6g | Protein 24.9g)

Creamy Zucchini Soup

(Total Time: 2 HR 20 MIN| **Serve:** 6)

Ingredients:

1 small onion, minced
4 cups grated zucchini with peel
2 cups chicken stock
1 tsp salt
1 tsp dried dill
1/2 tsp white pepper
2 Tbsp butter, melted
1 cup sour cream

Directions:

1. Mix together everything, except the sour cream, in a greased slow cooker.
2. Cook covered for 2 hours on low.
3. Mix in the sour cream and cook for an additional 10 minutes, or until heated through.
4. Ladle into bowls and enjoy!

(Calories 233 | Total Fats 8.5g | Net Carbs: 3.41g | Protein 34g)

Indian Curried Cauliflower Soup

(Total Time: 5 HR 15 MIN| Serve: 4)

Ingredients:

1 head cauliflower
2 cups chicken stock
3 cloves garlic
1 canned coconut milk
1 cup plain yogurt
1 Tbsp curry powder
Salt and pepper to taste
1/4 cup toasted pine nuts
3/4 tsp garam masala
1/2 cup xylitol
1/2 tsp salt
1 Tbsp water

Directions:

1. Cut cauliflower from the stalk, place in slow cooker, put chicken stock and garlic in the slow cooker.
2. Cover and cook until tender, about 2-4 hours on low.
3. Add coconut milk and yogurt to slow cooker and cook for an additional 1 hour on low, then using a hand blender, blend until pureed.
4. Sprinkle with toasted pine nuts and some fresh mint.

(Calories 219 | Total Fats 7g | Net Carbs: 4.13g | Protein 33.7g)

Broccoli & Blue cheese Soup

(Total Time: 4 HR 20 MIN| **Serve:** 6)

Ingredients:

2 onion, diced

4 stick celery, sliced

4 leek, sliced (white part only)

2 Tbsp butter

4 cups chicken stock

2 large heads of broccoli, cut into florets

1 1/4 cups crumbled blue cheese

1/2 cup cream

Directions:

1. Put all of the ingredients into your slow cooker.
2. Stir to combine.
3. Put the lid on the slow cooker and cook on high for 4 hours (or 8 hours on low).
4. Using a hand blender, blitz the soup until smooth
5. Ladle into bowls and top with extra crumbles of blue cheese (if desired).

(Calories 174 | Total Fats 10g | Net Carbs: 12.8g | Protein 7.5g)

Italian Meatball Zoodle Soup

(Total Time: 6 HR 45 MIN| Serve: 6)

Ingredients:

32 oz. beef stock
1 medium zucchini, spiraled
2 ribs celery, chopped
1 small onion, diced
1 carrot, chopped
1 medium tomato, diced
1 ½ tsp garlic salt
1 ½ lb. ground beef
½ cup parmesan cheese, shredded
6 cloves garlic, minced
1 egg
4 Tbsp fresh parsley, chopped
1 ½ tsp sea salt
1 ½ tsp onion powder
1 tsp Italian seasoning
1 tsp dried oregano
½ tsp black pepper

Directions:

1. Heat slow cooker on low setting.
2. Add zucchini, celery, tomato, carrot onion, beef stock and garlic salt to the slow cooker. Cover.
3. In a large bowl, combine together Italian seasoning, oregano, onion powder, sea salt, parsley, egg, garlic, parmesan, ground beef, and pepper.
4. Using mixture, make approximately 30 meatballs by rolling with your hands.
5. Heat olive oil in a large skillet over medium-high heat.
6. Once the pan is hot, add meatballs and brown on all sides.
7. Add meatballs into the slow cooker, cover with a lid and cook for 6 hours, before serving.

(Calories 352 | Total Fats 19g | Net Carbs: 4.5g | Protein 40g)

BBQ Chicken Soup

(Total Time: 1 HR 50 MIN| **Serve:** 4)

Ingredients:

For Soup Base:
3 chicken thighs
Salt
1 ½ cups chicken broth
2 tsp chili seasoning
2 Tbsp olive oil
1 ½ cups beef broth
Black pepper

For BBQ Sauce:
¼ cup ketchup
2 Tbsp Dijon mustard
1 Tbsp hot sauce
1 tsp Worcestershire sauce
1 tsp onion powder
1 tsp red chili flakes
¼ cup butter
¼ cup tomato paste
1 Tbsp soy sauce
2 ½ tsp liquid smokes
1 ½ tsp garlic powder
1 tsp chili powder
1 tsp cumin

Directions:

1. Set oven to 400 F. Remove bones from chicken and put bones aside. Season chicken with chili seasoning and place into oven for 50 minutes.
2. Heat oil in a deep pot and add bones. Cook for 5 minutes then add beef and chicken broth; season with pepper and salt.

3. Take chicken from oven and remove skin. Add the fat to the soup and mix together. Combine BBQ sauce ingredients and add to pot. Cook for 30 minutes.
4. Combine fats in the soup by using an immersion blender, then shred chicken and add to soup. Cook for 20 minutes.
5. Serve topped with chicken skin. May add cheese or bell peppers.

(Calories 487 | Total Fats 38.3g | Net Carbs: 4.3g | Protein 24.5g)

Super-Fast Egg Drop Soup

(Total Time: 15 MIN| Serve: 1)

Ingredients:

1 ½ cups chicken broth
1 Tbsp butter
1 tsp chili garlic paste
½ cube chicken bouillon
2 eggs

Directions:

1. Add butter to pan, heat until it melts, then add broth and bouillon
2. Bring to a boil and add chili paste, stir to combine and remove fromheat.
3. Beat eggs in a bowl and add to broth, stir and put aside for a few minutes.
4. Serve.

(Calories 279 | Total Fats 23g | Net Carbs: 2.5g | Protein 12g)

Spicy Slow-Cooked Chicken Soup

(Total Time: 6 HR 10 MIN| Serve: 4)

Ingredients:

4 boneless chicken fillets
4 bacon strips
1 small onion, sliced thin
1 bell pepper, sliced thin
½ Tbsp fresh thyme
½ Tbsp garlic, minced
½ Tbsp coconut flour
½ cup low-sodium chicken stock
¼ cup coconut milk, unsweetened
1 ½ Tbsp tomato paste
1 ½ Tbsp lemon juice
1 Tbsp butter
Salt and pepper to taste

Directions:

1. Place the butter in the middle of the slow cooker.
2. Add the onion and bell pepper slices at the bottom and then top with the chicken fillets.
3. Chop the bacon and sprinkle on top of the chicken.
4. Add the rest of the ingredients (liquids last) and then cover and cook on low for 6 hours.
5. Uncover after 6 hours and break the chicken up into smaller pieces before serving.
6. Serve with a spoonful of sour cream on top.

(Calories 396 | Total Fats 21g | Net Carbs: 7g | Protein 41g)

BBQ Pizza Soup

(Total Time: 25 MIN| **Serve: 8**)

Ingredients:

6 chicken legs
4 garlic cloves
4 cups green beans
1 ½ cups mozzarella cheese
12 cups water
½ tsp black pepper
1 red onion (chopped)
14 oz. canned tomatoes (sugar-free)
¾ cup BBQ sauce
¼ cup ghee
1 tsp salt
Basil (chopped)

Directions:

1. Add water and salt to a pot and boil chicken for 60 minutes (or more), until meat is falling off bones. Shred chicken and put aside until needed.
2. Heat ghee in a soup pot and sauté garlic and onion until golden and aromatic. Add broth from boiling chicken by straining into the pot.
3. Clean and chop beans and add to pot along with tomatoes. Cook for 15 minutes.
4. Add shredded chicken and BBQ sauce and remove from flame. Add pepper and salt to taste.
5. Top with mozzarella cheese, stir and ladle into bowls.
6. Serve topped with basil.

(Calories 449 | Total Fats 32.5g | Net Carbs: 10g | Protein 30.8g)

Cheese and Bacon Soup

(Total Time: 30 MIN| Serve: 4)

Ingredients:

3 bacon strips, cooked and chopped
1 cup cheddar, shredded
1 cup Monterey jack cheese, shredded
1 small bell pepper, chopped
2 cloves of garlic, minced
1 onion, chopped fine
12 oz. gluten-free beer
½ cup milk
½ cup light cream
2 Tbsp butter
2 Tbsp flour
Salt and pepper to taste

Directions:

1. Using the grease from cooking bacon, sauté the onions and bell pepper for 5 minutes in a pot over medium heat.
2. Adjust the heat to low and add the garlic and cook for another 2 minutes.
3. Increase the heat again and then add the 2 Tbsp butter and allow it to boil.
4. Add the 2 Tbsp flour to the pot and whisk for 3 minutes.
5. Pour the beer and stir constantly for 5 minutes.
6. Lower the heat again and add the milk and light cream.
7. Remove the pot from the heat and then add the cheese. Stir until the cheese has completely melted.
8. Season with salt and pepper and transfer into serving bowls.
9. Garnish with crispy bacon on top. Serve hot.

(Calories 442 | Total Fats 34g | Net Carbs: 11g | Protein 20g)

Beef Cabbage Parsley Soup

(Total Time: 2 HR 5 MIN| Serve: 8)

Ingredients:

1 lb. beef shank
1/2 head cabbage, chopped
6 tsp fresh parsley (chopped)
2 zucchini, cubed
1 tomato, quartered
1 onion, chopped
4 cloves garlic, minced
1 Tbsp salt
1/4 tsp ground cumin
2 Tbsp fresh lime juice

Directions:

1. In a large pot over low heat, combine the beef, tomato, zucchini, onion, cabbage, garlic, 5 tsp parsley, salt, and cumin.
2. Add water to cover and stir well. Cover the lid and cook for 2 hours.
3. Remove lid, stir, and simmer for another 1 hour with lid off.
4. Just before eating, squeeze in fresh lime juice to taste and sprinkle with remaining parsley.
5. Serve hot.

(Calories 129 | Total Fats 2.3g | Net Carbs: 13.2g | Protein 14.1g)

Boneless Lamb Stew

(Total Time: 2 HR 10 MIN| Serve: 6)

Ingredients:

2 lbs. boneless lamb meat, cubed
1 cup red onion, chopped
2 whole celery stalks, diced
4 cloves garlic, minced
1 cup tomato juice
2 Tbsp extra virgin coconut oil
1 cup lime juice (freshly squeezed)
1 bay leaf
1 tsp ground cinnamon
1 tsp ground nutmeg
Fresh parsley, chopped for topping
Sea salt and freshly ground black pepper, to taste

Directions:

1. Put the lamb in a glass bowl and season with the salt, pepper, cinnamon, and nutmeg. Place in refrigerator for up to 24 hours.
2. In a large casserole, heat the coconut oil over medium heat. Add pieces of lamb and brown on all sides.
3. Once browned, add the onion, garlic, and celery. Cook for about five minutes, stirring often until vegetables start to soften.
4. Add the tomato juice, lime juice, and bay leaf; stir till mixture begins to boil.
5. Reduce the heat to low and cook for about 2 hours.
6. Serve hot with fresh chopped parsley.

(Calories 250 | Total Fats 11.8g | Net Carbs: 6.8g | Protein 21g)

Keto Butternut Squash Soup

(Total Time: 55 MIN| **Serve:** 10)

Ingredients:

3 lbs. butternut squash
4 cloves garlic, minced
1 cup yellow onion, sliced
1 cup coconut milk
2 tsp olive oil
1 bay leaf
2 cup water
1/2 tsp salt and pepper (per taste)
Coconut oil or olive oil for greasing

Directions:

1. Preheat oven to 450 F.
2. On a greased baking sheet, place the squash and onion with half oil and salt. Roast in a single layer about 25-30 minutes.
3. Transfer the vegetables to a large saucepan with olive oil and cook over HIGH heat for 3-5 minutes. Stir often.
4. Add garlic and cook for another 30 seconds. Add the water, bay leaf, and coconut milk; bring to a boil.
5. Reduce heat to Medium Low, cover and simmer for 10 minutes more.
6. At the end, remove bay leaf and transfer squash mixture to a blender. Puree until smooth. Add salt and pepper to taste.
7. Ladle into bowls and serve hot.

(Calories 120 | Total Fats 7.2g | Net Carbs: 12.7g | Protein 3.4g)

Spinach Soup with Almonds and Parmesan

(Total Time: 45 MIN| Serve: 6)

Ingredients:

1 lb. baby spinach leaves
1 leek
1 zucchini (medium)
1/4 cup parmesan cheese (grated)
4 Tbsp olive oil
4 cups water
15 almond slivers
Salt and black ground pepper to taste

Directions:

1. Wash the leek and cut it into thick slices.
2. Heat the olive oil in a saucepan and cook the zucchini and leek for about 2-3 minutes.
3. Add the cleaned spinach leaves, water and a pinch of salt. Bring to the boil and let it simmer for 15 minutes.
4. Remove from the heat and place the vegetables in a food processor. Blend into a very smooth soup.
5. In a frying pan, toast the almonds. Pour the soup into bowls, sprinkle with some Parmesan cheese on top and toasted almonds.
6. Serve.

(Calories 63.4 | Total Fats 3.4g | Net Carbs: 5.9g | Protein 4.84g)

Keto Light Cabbage Soup

(Total Time: 35 MIN| Serve: 4)

Ingredients:

2 1/2 cups chopped cabbage
4 garlic cloves, minced
1 Tbsp tomato paste
1 onion, chopped
1/2 cup parsnip, chopped
1/2 cup cauliflower florets
1/2 cup chopped zucchini
1/2 tsp basil
1/2 tsp oregano
Salt and black pepper, to taste
4 cups water
Olive oil for sautéing

Directions:

1. In a frying pan, sauté onions, parsnip, and garlic for 5 minutes.
2. Add in water, tomato paste, cabbage, cauliflower, basil, oregano and salt and pepper to taste.
3. Simmer for about 5-10 minutes until all vegetables are tender. Add the zucchini and simmer for another 5 minutes.
4. Serve hot.

(Calories 80.31| Total Fats 3.8g | Net Carbs: 9.69g | Protein 4.62g)

Oriental Shrimp Soup

(Total Time: 25 MIN| Serve: 8)

Ingredients:

12 oz. fresh shrimp, peeled and deveined
1 cup zucchini (medium, sliced)
1 onion, chopped
2 cloves garlic, minced
1 Tbsp ginger, minced
1 pinch crushed red pepper
2 quarts water
1 cup celery (chopped)
2 cups cauliflower florets
2 Tbsp soy sauce
1/4 tsp ground black pepper
2 tsp olive oil

Directions:

1. In a large saucepan with over medium heat, cook onion, garlic, ginger and crushed red pepper for 2 minutes.
2. Pour in water, cauliflower florets, and celery and bring to a boil. Reduce heat, cover and simmer 5 minutes.
3. Stir in zucchini and shrimp, season with salt and pepper to taste; cover and cook 5 - 7 minutes.
4. Stir in soy sauce and pepper and serve.

(Calories 107.62 | Total Fats 3.08g | Net Carbs: 7.12g | Protein 12.08g)

Zucchini Soup with Crunchy Cured Ham

(Total Time: 45 MIN| Serve: 4)

Ingredients:

2 leeks (white part only)
12 ounces zucchini
10 ounces summer squash
3 Tbsp extra virgin olive oil
5 cups water
Salt
2 slices cured ham
Black pepper

Directions:

1. Cut the leeks into thin slices and chop the zucchini and summer squash into cubes.
2. In a large saucepan, heat the olive oil and add the leeks. Cook the leeks until they are soft, stirring gently.
3. Add in the chopped zucchini and summer squash and cook them for about 5 minutes.
4. Add in water and bring to the boil for about 15 minutes.
5. Blend or process the soup in batches until smooth.
6. Season the soup to taste.
7. In a frying pan cook striped ham until crispy.
8. Divide the soup amongst the serving bowls and sprinkle with the crunchy ham strips and some black pepper.
9. Serve hot.

(Calories 84.19 | Total Fats 31.7g | Net Carbs: 8.75g | Protein 854g)

Hot Chili Soup

(Total Time: 45 MIN| Serve: 4)

Ingredients:

1 tsp coriander seeds
2 chili pepper, sliced
2 cups water
½ tsp ground cumin
16 oz chicken thighs
1 avocado
4 Tbsp cilantro, chopped
Salt
2 Tbsp olive oil
2 cups chicken broth
1 tsp turmeric
4 Tbsp tomato paste
2 Tbsp butter
2 oz queso fresco
Lime juice freshly squeezed
Black pepper

Directions:

1. Chop chicken thighs and heat oil in a soup pot. Add chicken to the pot and cook for 8 minutes, then remove from pot and put aside.
2. Add coriander to the pot and cook until aromatic, then add chili and cook for 1 minute.
3. Add water and broth and bring mixture to a boil. Add cumin, turmeric, black pepper and salt to taste.
4. When soup starts to boil, add butter and tomato paste, stir until butter melts and the mixture is thoroughly combined. Cook for 10 minutes then adds lime juice.
5. Add cooked chicken to soup and cook for 5 minutes.
6. Serve topped with queso fresco and avocado.

(Calories 396 | Total Fats 27.8g | Net Carbs: 5.8g | Protein 28g)

Jalapeno Popper Soup

(Total Time: 1 HR 30 MIN| Serve: 6)

Ingredients:

Salt
Black pepper
3 jalapenos, diced
1 tsp onion powder
1 tsp cajun seasoning
3 cups chicken broth
4 oz cheddar cheese
4 chicken thighs, bones removed
1 Tbsp chicken fat
2 tsp garlic, diced
1 tsp cilantro, dried
6 oz cream cheese
4 bacon slices

Directions:

1. Set oven to 400 F.
2. Remove bones from thighs, season with pepper and salt and bake for 55 minutes.
3. Heat pot and heat 1 tbsp chicken fat, then add bones to pot; fry for 10 minutes.
4. Add garlic and jalapeno, cook for 4 minutes until vegetables are softened.
5. Add spice to pot, stir and add broth, scraping pan to remove bits and cook until chicken is thoroughly cooked. Take skins from thighs and take bones from broth.
6. Add remaining fat to the pot along with garlic and jalapenos and use an immersion blender to puree mixture. Shred chicken and put into the pot, cook for 15 minutes then add cheddar and cream cheese. Cook for 5 minutes, until cheese melts.
7. Heat skillet and cook bacon until crisp. Cool and crumble bacon.
8. Serve soup with bacon on top and chicken skins.

(Calories 550 | Total Fats 42.7g | Net Carbs: 3g | Protein 33.7g)

Cheeseburger Soup

(Total Time: 40 MIN| Serve: 5)

Ingredients:

12 oz ground beef
3 cups beef broth
½ tsp onion powder
1 ½ tsp kosher salt
½ tsp red pepper flakes
1 tsp chili powder
1 dill pickle, diced
3 oz cream cheese
5 bacon slices
2 Tbsp butter
½ tsp garlic powder
2 tsp brown mustard
½ tsp black pepper
1 tsp Cumin
2 ½ Tbsp tomato paste
1 cup cheddar cheese, shredded
½ cup heavy cream

Directions:

1. Heat pan and cook bacon until crisp, remove from pot and put aside until needed.
2. Add beef to pot and cook for 10 minutes, until browned all over.
3. Transfer beef to a soup pot, add butter to the soup pot along with spices and cook for 45 seconds. Then add tomato paste, pickles, beef broth and cheese, cook for 3 minutes until melted.
4. Lower heat and cook for 30 minutes.
5. Remove from heat and add bacon and cream, stir and serve.

(Calories 572 | Total Fats 48.6g | Net Carbs: 3.4g | Protein 23.4g)

Malaysian Bone Broth Soup

(Total Time: 1 HR 10 MIN| Serve: 5)

Ingredients:

2 lb pork ribs, cut into cubes
1 whole garlic, crushed
1 cup dried shiitake mushrooms
1 cup enoki mushrooms
2 sachets Bak Kuh Teh
Pepper to taste
12 cups water

Directions:

1. Bring the water to a boil, with the Bak Kuh Teh sachets in it.
2. When boiling, place the ribs in the pot and reduce the heat.
3. Throw the crushed garlic into the pot and then add the mushrooms. Stir.
4. Cook for 1 hour or a few minutes more.
5. Serve hot.

(Calories 517 | Total Fats 32.2g | Net Carbs: 5.0g | Protein 48.8g)

Cheeseburger Soup Indulgence

(Total Time: 40 MIN| Serve: 5)

Ingredients:

5 strips of bacon, cooked and crumbled

12 oz ground beef

3 cups beef broth

2 Tbsp organic butter

½ tsp onion powder

½ tsp garlic powder

2 tsp Dijon mustard

1 ½ tsp salt

½ tsp pepper

½ tsp red pepper flakes

1 tsp cumin

1 tsp chili powder

2 ½ Tbsp tomato paste

¼ cup pickles, diced

1 cup cheddar cheese, shredded

¼ cream cheese

½ cup heavy cream

Directions:

1. Using the same pan where the bacon was cooked, add the ground beef and cook until done.
2. Place the browned beef into a pot and add the butter and the spices. Cook for 45 seconds.
3. Pour in the beef broth, cheddar, tomato paste, diced pickles and cook until the cheese melts.
4. Cover the pot and cook for 30minutes on low heat.
5. Turn off the heat and add the heavy cream and cream cheese on top and garnish with the bacon.

(Calories 572 | Total Fats 3.4g | Net Carbs: 3.4g | Protein 23.4g)

Cabbage with Ground Beef Stew

(Total Time: 25 MIN| Serve: 10)

Ingredients:

1 1/2 lb. ground beef
2 lbs. green cabbage
1/2 cup unsalted butter
1/2 cup water
3 cups pasta sauce
Salt and pepper to taste

Directions:

1. In a food processor, shred quartered cabbage.
2. In a saucepan, melt the butter and add the cabbage, water and salt and pepper to taste.
3. Cover and cook for 12-15 minutes, stirring occasionally
4. In a meanwhile, in a frying pan brown the ground beef.
5. Once browned, add the beef to the cabbage and stir well. Finally, add the pasta sauce and stir. Serve hot.

(Calories 307 | Total Fats 22g | Net Carbs: 12.3g | Protein 14.9g)

Slow Cooker Roast and Chicken Stew

(Total Time: 8 HR 10 MIN| Serve: 10)

Ingredients:

3 lb. pot roast

1 lb. chicken breast (boiled and shredded)

6 oz. Italian sweet sausage

2 cups beef broth

1 cup chicken stock

1/2 medium onion (chopped)

1 can (11 oz.) low-carb diced tomatoes

1/4 tsp thyme

1/4 tsp celery salt

1 Tbsp coconut oil

1 tsp basil

2 tsp dried dill weed

2 tsp garlic powder

2 tsp pepper

1 Tbsp garlic salt

1 tsp minced garlic

1 Tbsp oregano

1 Tbsp powdered buttermilk

4 tsp onion powder

4 tsp dried parsley

5 tsp red pepper flakes

2 tsp hot sauce

Directions:

1. At the bottom of your slow cooker, place roast, chicken breast, and Italian sausages. Add on the top all other ingredients and stir lightly.
2. Close the lid and cook on Low for about 6-8 hours.
3. Once ready, flavor to taste with some additional hot sauce, salt, and pepper to your own liking and serve hot.

(Calories 467 | Total Fats 36g | Net Carbs: 3.7g | Protein 30g)

Italian Fish Stew

(Total Time: 55 MIN| **Serve:** 4)

Ingredients:

4 kingklip fish fillets
2 onions, finely chopped
4 garlic cloves, minced
2 tins peeled, chopped tomato
4 Tbsp tomato paste
1 cup white wine
½ tsp parsley, chopped
¼ tsp dried oregano
Salt and pepper to taste
½ cup olive oil
1 cup water

Directions:

1. Preheat oven to 680 F.
2. Sauté onion and garlic in a pot, then add tinned tomatoes and tomato paste and stir.
3. Pour the wine, parsley, oregano, salt, pepper, and water. Stir well and bring to a simmer.
4. Let it simmer for 10-15 minutes to reduce and thicken.
5. Meanwhile, place your fish in baking dish.
6. When the sauce is nice and thick, pour it over fish and sprinkle with a little extra oregano.
7. Cover the dish with foil and place in the oven to cook for 20 minutes.
8. Take foil off and return to oven uncovered and cook for another 10 minutes.

(Calories 315 | Total Fats 8g | Net Carbs: 12g | Protein 37g)

Chicken and Mushroom Stew

(Total Time: 45 MIN| Serve: 10)

Ingredients:

8 pcs chicken thighs
4 Tbsp butter
3 cloves garlic, minced
6 cups mushrooms
1 cup chicken stock
½ tsp dried thyme
½ tsp dried oregano
½ tsp dried basil
¼ cup heavy cream
½ cup parmesan cheese, grated
1 Tbsp whole-grain mustard

Directions:

1. Preheat oven to 400 F.
2. Season chicken thighs with salt and pepper.
3. Heat an oven-proof pan over the medium fire and melt 2 Tbsp of butter.
4. Add the chicken, skin-side down, and fry both sides until golden brown, or about 2-3 minutes per side. Set aside.
5. Melt remaining 2 Tbsp butter. Add garlic, thyme, oregano and basil and mushrooms, and cook, stirring occasionally. Cook until browned, about 5-6 minutes, season with salt and pepper, to taste.
6. Stir in chicken stock, then chicken back to the pan.
7. Pour everything into a baking dish with the chicken.
8. Place into oven and roast until completely cooked through for about 25-30 minutes. Set aside chicken.
9. Transfer sauces back into the original pan.
10. Stir in heavy cream, parmesan cheese, and mustard. Bring to a boil; reduce heat and simmer until slightly reduced about 5 minutes.
11. Serve chicken immediately, topped with mushroom mixture.

(Calories 203 | Total Fats 3g | Net Carbs: 9g | Protein 28g)

Beef Shin Stew

(Total Time: 3 HR 25 MIN| Serve: 8)

Ingredients:

2 lb. quality shin of beef, cubed

4 tbsp olive oil

2 red onions, peeled and roughly chopped

3 carrots, peeled and roughly chopped

3 sticks celery, trimmed and roughly chopped

4 cloves garlic, unpeeled

a few sprigs of fresh rosemary

2 bay leaves

2 cups mushrooms

2 cups baby marrows

Salt and pepper to taste

1 Tbsp psyllium husk

2 cans tomatoes

⅔ bottle red wine

Directions:

1. Preheat your oven to 360 F.
2. In a heavy-bottomed oven-proof saucepan, heat olive oil and sauté the onions, carrots, celery, garlic, herbs, and mushrooms for 5 minutes until softened slightly.
3. Meanwhile, roll the beef in psyllium husk.
4. Then add meat into saucepan and stir until all ingredients are mixed.
5. Add the tomatoes, wine and a pinch of salt and pepper and gently bring to the boil.
6. Once boiling, turn off the heat and cover the saucepan with double thickness tinfoil and the lid.
7. Place saucepan in the oven to cook and develop flavor for 3 hours or until the beef can be pulled apart with a spoon.
8. Taste and add more salt if necessary.
9. Serve and enjoy.

(Calories 315 | Total Fats 7g | Net Carbs: 7g | Protein 20g)

Tuna Fish Stew

(Total Time: 25 MIN| Serve: 2)

Ingredients:

1 tin tuna in water, drained
1 Tbsp butter
¼ small onion, chopped finely
1 clove garlic, minced
1 tsp fresh ginger, grated
½ tin tomatoes, chopped finely
1 cup spinach, chopped finely
1 small carrot, grated
1 tsp curry powder
 1 tsp turmeric
½ tsp cayenne pepper (optional)
Salt & pepper to taste

Directions:

1. Fry onion, garlic, and ginger in butter.
2. Add tomatoes once onions are soft.
3. Add enough water to make a stew for the spinach, carrot and tuna fish. Cook at low heat for about 15 minutes(Do not overcook spinach).
4. Steam 2 cups of cauliflower, mash and add 1Tblsp of butter. Serve stew on top of the caulimash.

(Calories 253 | Total Fats 5g | Net Carbs: 7g | Protein 25g)

Cauliflower and Cheese Chowder

(Total Time: 30 MIN| **Serve:** 4)

Ingredients:

4 cups cauliflower florets, chopped
4 bacon strips
1 Tbsp organic butter
2 cloves of garlic, minced
1 onion, chopped fine
¼ cup almond flour
4 cups low-sodium chicken broth
½ cup milk
¼ cup light cream
1 cup cheddar, shredded
Salt and pepper to taste

Directions:

1. Cook the bacon in a large pot. Remove from the pot when cooked and set aside.
2. Using the same pot set the heat on medium and throw in the onions. Cook for 3 minutes and then add the garlic and cauliflower florets and cook for another 5 minutes.
3. Add the flour into the pot and continuously whisk for a minute.
4. Pour the chicken broth, milk, and light cream and stir for 3 minutes.
5. Allow to simmer for 15 minutes and then turn off the heat.
6. Add the cheddar cheese into the pot, season with salt and pepper and stir again.
7. Serve with the chopped bacon on top.

(Calories 268 | Total Fats 15.9g | Net Carbs: 11.9g | Protein 19.5g)

Chicken Bacon Chowder

(Total Time: 8 HR s10 MIN| **Serve:** 5)

Ingredients:

4 cloves garlic – minced

1 leek – cleaned, trimmed, and sliced

2 ribs celery – diced

1 punnet button mushrooms – sliced

2 medium sweet onion – thinly sliced

4 Tbsp butter

2 cups chicken stock

6 boneless, skinless chicken breasts, butterflied

8 oz. cream cheese

1 cup heavy cream

1 packet streaky bacon – cooked crisp, and crumbled

1 tsp salt

1 tsp pepper

1 tsp garlic powder

1 tsp thyme

Directions:

1. Select low setting on your slow cooker.
2. Place 1 cup of chicken stock, onions, garlic, mushroom, leeks, celery, 2 Tbsp of butter, and the salt and pepper into your slow cooker.
3. Put the lid on, and cook ingredients on low for 1 hour.
4. Brown chicken breasts in a skillet with 2 Tbsp of butter.
5. Add the remaining 1 cup of chicken stock.
6. Scrape the bottom of the skillet to remove any chicken that may have stuck to the bottom.
7. Remove from skillet and set aside, pouring the fat from the pan over the chicken.
8. Add in the thyme, heavy cream, garlic powder and cream cheese into your slow cooker.
9. Stir the contents of the slow cooker until the cream cheese has melted into the dish.
10. Cut the chicken into cubes. Add the bacon and chicken cubes into the slow cooker. Stir ingredients and cook on low for 6-8 hours.

(Calories 355 | Total Fats 21g | Net Carbs: 6.4g | Protein 28g)

Chapter 9: Vegetable Recipes

Squash Carbonara

(Total Time: 25 MIN| Serve: 3)

Ingredients:

1 pack konjac yam noodles (Shirataki)
2 egg yolks
3 Tbsp squash puree
1/3 cup parmesan cheese, grated
½ cup heavy cream
2 Tbsp organic butter
4 pcs pancetta
½ tsp dried sage
Salt and pepper to taste

Directions:

1. Boil water and soak the noodles in it for 3 minutes. Strain and set aside.
2. Sear the pancetta on a hot pan, and chop. Reserve the fat from the pancetta.
3. Place the strained noodles on the pan cooked for the pancetta and cook for 5 minutes. Set aside.
4. On another pan (large sized) melt the butter on medium heat and allow to brown. Add the squash puree and season with sage.
5. Pour the heavy cream into the pan, add the fat from the pancetta and stir well.
6. Lastly, add the parmesan cheese into the sauce and the mix well. Reduce the heat to low and stir until the sauce thickens.
7. Transfer the noodles into the pan with the sauce, crack the eggs and combine all the ingredients together.

(Calories 384 | Total Fats 34.7g | Net Carbs: 2g | Protein 14g)

Ratatouille

(Total Time: 20 MIN| Serve: 4)

Ingredients:

2 large brinjals
1 large onion
2 peppers (can be green, red, and yellow)
2 tins of chopped tomatoes
1 packet baby marrows
1 punnet mushrooms
1 packet spinach
2 ¼ cups chicken stock
Salt & pepper
2 cloves garlic (finely chopped or pressed)

To serve:
150g chunky cottage cheese/30g cheddar or 6 Tbsp parmesan cheese

Directions:

1. Finely chop all the ingredients.
2. Add all the finely chopped veggies, garlic, and onion to the stock and boil on medium until the water has reduced, and the veggies have formed a thick delicious stew.
3. Serve with your choice of cheese.

(Calories 149 | Total Fats 2g | Net Carbs: 29g | Protein 7g)

Cauliflower Bake

(Total Time: 40 MIN| Serve: 10)

Ingredients:

4 slices of bacon
2 cups broccoli
2 cups cauliflower
2 cups mushrooms
1 green pepper
1 onion
1 cup cream
3 Tbsp cheddar cheese, grated
2 Tbsp olive oil

Directions:

1. Preheat oven to 360 F.
2. Steam or cook the cauliflower and broccoli until tender then transfer to an oven-proof dish.
3. Fry the bacon slices, with the mushrooms, green pepper, and onion in 2 tbsp olive oil.
4. Pour the fried bacon and mushrooms on top of cauliflower.
5. In a bowl, whisk 4 eggs with the cream and season to taste and pour over cauliflower or broccoli.
6. Place in the oven to cook for 25 minutes. Take out of the oven and sprinkle with grated cheese.
7. Place back in the oven and cook for another 5 minutes, before serving.

(Calories 100 | Total Fats 6g | Net Carbs: 7g| Protein 4g)

Caulicake

(Total Time: 55 MIN| Serve: 10)

Ingredients:

1.3 lbs cauliflower florets

1 onion, chopped

3 cloves of garlic, finely chopped

1 tsp turmeric

1 cup parmesan cheese, finely grated

1 cup mature white cheddar cheese, coarsely grated

8 eggs

1-2 tsp salt

2 Tbsp psyllium husk

1 cup of cream

1 Tbsp coconut oil

Sesame seeds

Olive oil

Directions:

1. Preheat oven to 360 F.
2. Steam the cauliflower. Keep half of it whole and mash the rest.
3. Sauté the onion, garlic, turmeric in the coconut oil until soft. Set aside.
4. In a separate bowl, whisk the eggs. Add the cream, cheese, salt, and psyllium husk.
5. Combine the cauliflower, whole and mashed with the sautéed onions and egg mixture in a bowl.
6. Line a spring-form baking tin with greased baking paper and sprinkle with sesame seeds. Place the pan onto a baking tray.
7. Pour in the cauliflower mix and bake in the oven for 40 minutes.
8. As soon as it comes out of the oven, lightly prick the surface all over with a fork and drizzle with olive oil.
9. Serve and enjoy!

(Calories 160 | Total Fats 11g | Net Carbs: 5g | Protein 8g)

Spiced Kale "Meatballs"

(Total Time: 25 MIN| **Serve:** 8)

Ingredients:

4 Tbsp olive oil
1 cup almond flour
1 bunch of kale leaves
1 green chili, chopped
1/4 tsp red chili powder
1/4 tsp turmeric powder
1 tsp cumin seed powder
1/4 tsp ginger, minced
Black salt or salt as per taste
1 tsp cooking soda or baking soda (optional)
Water for batter

Directions:

1. In a bowl, mix all the ingredients together.
2. Combine and knead the batter with your fingers. The consistency should be not too thick nor too thin. Make kale "meatballs".
3. Heat oil in a frying pan. Place a kale "meatballs" in the hot oil, one by one.
4. Fry few at a time, don't cluster with too many. When they get golden color on one side, turn and cook on another side.
5. Remove the fries with slotted spoon and place over absorbent napkins.
6. Serve hot.

(Calories 125 | Total Fats 6.2g | Net Carbs: 13g | Protein 6g)

Pumpkin Carbonara

(Total Time: 30 MIN| Serve: 4)

Ingredients:

5 oz pancetta
¼ cup heavy cream
2 Tbsp butter
½ tsp sage, dried
Black pepper
1 packet Shirataki noodles
2 egg yolks
1/3 cup parmesan cheese
3 Tbsp pumpkin puree
Salt

Directions:

1. Boil a pot of water and add noodles, cook for 3 minutes then drain. Dry completely and put aside until needed.
2. Chop pancetta, heat skillet and cook pancetta until crispy. Reserve oil and put pancetta aside, until needed.
3. Heat a small pot and add butter, cook, until it gets brown then add puree and sage.
4. Add pancetta, fat and cream, mix together until thoroughly combined.
5. Heat pan that had in fat on a high flame and stirs fry noodles for 5 minutes.
6. Add cheese to pumpkin mixture, combine and lower heat; cook until sauce gets thick.
7. Add pancetta and noodles to sauce, toss before adding yolks and mix together; cook for 3 minutes.
8. Serve.

(Calories 384 | Total Fats 34.7g | Net Carbs: 2g | Protein 14g)

One Pot Italian Sausage Meal

(Total Time: 25 MIN| Serve: 2)

Ingredients:

1 Tbsp onion
¼ cup parmesan cheese
½ tsp oregano
¼ tsp salt
3 sausage links
4 oz. mushrooms
¼ cup mozzarella cheese (shredded)
½ tsp basil
¼ tsp red pepper flakes

Directions:

1. Set oven to 350 F.
2. Heat a cast iron skillet until it starts to smoke, then add sausages and cook until almost done.
3. Slice onion and mushrooms and remove sausages from the pot. Add sliced veggies and cook for 3 minutes until golden.
4. Slice sausages and add to skillet, along with seasonings. Add parmesan and stir to combine.
5. Place skillet into the oven and cook for 10 minutes, then top with mozzarella and cook until cheese melts.
6. Serve hot.

(Calories 500 | Total Fats 38g | Net Carbs: 4.5g | Protein 30g)

No-Sweat Spinach Salad

(Total Time: 15 MIN| Serve: 4)

Ingredients:

4 cups baby spinach
4 strips of bacon, cooked and crumbled
4 Tbsp blue cheese, crumbled
¼ cup macadamia nuts, chopped
½ onion, sliced thin
¼ cup vinaigrette

Directions:

1. Clean the baby spinach thoroughly and dry.
2. Place in a salad bowl.
3. Sprinkle the blue cheese, bacon, and nuts on top.
4. Add the onions and then drizzle with vinaigrette.
5. Serve alone as a light keto lunch.

(Calories 690 | Total Fats 66.9g | Net Carbs: 16.5g | Protein 13.9g)

Baked Cheesy Zucchini

(Total Time: 40 MIN| Serve: 2)

Ingredients:

2 zucchini, peeled and grated
¼ cup parmesan cheese, grated
½ cup mozzarella cheese, grated
1 clove of garlic
2 organic eggs
3 Tbsp organic butter, (separate 1 Tbsp)
1 tsp salt

Directions:

1. Place the grated zucchini in a bowl and season with salt. Let them rest for 25 minutes.
2. Set oven to 400 F.
3. After the zucchini has rested for 25 minutes, place it in the middle of a dishtowel and squeeze out the liquid. Set aside.
4. Heat the 2 Tbsp of butter in a pan and sauté the garlic for about a minute. Add the parmesan cheese and then throw the zucchini into the pan and cook for 6 minutes. Stir occasionally.
5. Transfer into an oven-safe dish and then sprinkle with the grated mozzarella.
6. Bake in the oven for 10 minutes or until the cheese has melted.
7. While waiting for the zucchini to bake, fry the eggs, using the remaining 1 Tbsp of butter.
8. Remove the zucchini from the oven when done baking and serve topped with the butter-fried egg.

(Calories 552 | Total Fats 42g | Net Carbs: 10g | Protein 37g)

Level-Up Spinach Salad

(Total Time: 25 MIN| **S**erve: 2)

Ingredients:

2 Tbsp organic butter

1 small onion, sliced thin

3 cups baby spinach

2 organic eggs, cooked hard boiled

2 bacon strips, cooked and chopped

4 Tbsp slivered almonds

4 Tbsp gorgonzola cheese

For the dressing

2 Tbsp extra virgin olive oil

2 Tbsp balsamic vinegar

Salt and pepper to taste

Directions:

1. Heat the butter in a pan over medium fire.
2. Add the onions, season with salt and pepper and cook for 15 minutes, or until the onions caramelize.
3. While waiting for the onions to cook, prepare the dressing by whisking all the ingredients in a bowl. Set aside.
4. Also prepare the salad by adding the spinach to the bowl and then top with the sliced hard-boiled eggs, cheese, almonds, caramelized onion, and bacon.
5. Drizzle with the dressing and toss to incorporate all the ingredients.

(Calories 607 | Total Fats 52g | Net Carbs: 13g | Protein 20g |)

Pizza in Mushroom Cups

(Total Time: 20 MIN| Serve: 3)

Ingredients:

3 large Portobello mushroom caps
3 tsp pizza seasoning
3 tomato, slices
½ cup fresh basil leaves, chopped
12 slices pepperoni
¼ cup mozzarella cheese
¼ cup cheddar cheese
¼ cup Monterey Jack
½ Tbsp olive oil

Directions:

1. Set the oven at 450 F.
2. Place the mushroom caps on a baking sheet lined with parchment paper and drizzle with olive oil.
3. Season with the pizza seasoning and top with the basil, tomato slices, cheeses, and season again.
4. Place in the oven to bake for 5-6 minutes, or until the cheese has melted.
5. Get the baking sheet out of the oven and then top with the pepperoni and place back in the oven and bake until the pepperoni is cooked.

(Calories 276| Total Fats 21g | Net Carbs: 6g | Protein 19g)

Hearty Salad

(Total Time: 10 MIN| Serve: 2)

Ingredients:

1 hard boiled egg, grated
2 slices of country ham, finely sliced
1.05 oz cheddar cheese
1 tomato, finely diced
2 Tbsp mayonnaise
1 cup finely sliced crispy lettuce
2 spring onions, finely chopped
½ green pepper, finely chopped

Directions:

1. Combine all the ingredients and then add the mayonnaise and mix gently to infuse flavors.
2. Serve as a light keto lunch.

(Calories 214 | Total Fats 14.6g | Net Carbs: 9.5g | Protein 12.2g)

Spinach and Goat Cheese Salad

(Total Time: 20 MIN| Serve: 2)

Ingredients:

4 cups spinach
4 strawberries
1 ½ cups goat cheese (grated)
½ cup almond flakes (toasted)
4 Tbsp vinaigrette

Directions:

1. Set oven to 400 F and use parchment paper to line a baking sheet. Cut paper in half.
2. Grate cheese onto sheet and form into circles.
3. Bake for 10 minutes until golden. Gently lift parchment paper and shape cheese around upside-down bowls, cool and remove.
4. Toss spinach with vinaigrette and place into a hardened cheese bowl. Top with almonds and strawberries And serve.

(Calories 645 | Total Fats 54.2g | Net Carbs: 9.8g | Protein 33.2g)

Greek Eggplant Salad

(Total Time: 1 HR 10 MIN| Serve: 6)

Ingredients:

2 lbs. eggplants
4 garlic cloves, crushed
Parsley, chopped
½ tsp salt
2.6 oz. onion, chopped
Lemon juice
¼ cup extra virgin olive oil

Directions:

1. Set oven to 350 F and rinse eggplants and pat dry, then place on a baking sheet.
2. Bake for 60 minutes, until soft.
3. Add onion to food processor and pulse until fine. Add oil to a bowl and transfer onion to a clean cloth or fine sieve, squeeze onion juice into the oil. Discard onion solids or save for future use.
4. Add garlic, parsley and lemon juice to bowl and whisk together.
5. When eggplants are cooled, slice and scoop insides into a bowl and mash. Add oil mixture to eggplants and stir. Add pepper and salt to taste.
6. Serve.

(Calories 130 | Total Fats 9.4g | Net Carbs: 12g | Protein 33.2g)

Egg and Avocado Salad

(Total Time: 15 MIN| Serve: 2)

Ingredients:

1 avocado, sliced
½ cup yogurt (full fat)
2 tsp Dijon mustard
4 eggs
4 cups mixed greens
2 garlic cloves (smashed)
Salt
Black pepper
Fresh herbs

Directions:

1. Cook eggs until hard-boiled and then place into a pan with cold water.
2. Prepare the dressing by mixing yogurt, mustard, and garlic together. Season with black pepper and salt.
3. Rinse and drain greens and place into a bowl.
4. Top with sliced avocados and slice eggs into quarters and also place on top of salad; drizzle with dressing, a dash of pepper and salt and serve.

(Calories 436 | Total Fats 36.3g | Net Carbs: 13.7g | Protein 17g)

Tricolor Salad

(Total Time: 10 MIN| Serve: 2)

Ingredients:

1 avocado
4.5 oz. mozzarella cheese
8 kalamata olives
2 Tbsp pesto
Salt
Black pepper
4 tomatoes
2 Tbsp olive oil (extra virgin)
Basil (chopped)

Directions:

1. Slice tomatoes and avocados. Remove seeds from olives and slice.
2. Add all sliced ingredients to a bowl and top with cheese, oil, and pesto.
3. Add pepper and salt to taste And aerve.

(Calories 581 | Total Fats 50.7g | Net Carbs: 17.6g | Protein 19.2g)

Cucumber Strawberry Salsa and Grilled Halloumi

(Total Time: 20 MIN| Serve: 4)

Ingredients:

14.1 oz. halloumi cheese
5.3 oz. cucumber
Lime juice (freshly squeezed from 1 lime)
1 Tbsp mint (chopped)
2 Tbsp olive oil (extra-virgin)
1 Tbsp butter
Black pepper
1 cup strawberries
1 jalapeno
1 garlic clove
2 Tbsp basil (chopped)
1 Tbsp balsamic vinegar
¼ tsp salt

Directions:

1. Chop strawberries, peel cucumber and dice; remove seeds from pepper and chop.
2. Chop herbs and crush garlic and add to a bowl. Add lime juice, vinegar, and oil and whisk together.
3. Add dressing to chopped vegetables and fruits, toss and add pepper and salt to taste.
4. Slice cheese, heat butter in a skillet and cook for 3 minutes until golden on each side.
5. Top grilled cheese with salsa and serve.

(Calories 449 | Total Fats 37.7g | Net Carbs: 8.1g | Protein 20.8g)

Green Veggie Salad

(Total Time: 10 MIN| Serve: 6)

Ingredients:

1 cup green beans, steamed lightly
1 cup broccoli florets, steamed lightly
1 small tomato, finely sliced
1 cup lettuce
1 round feta
¼ cup toasted sunflower seeds, roasted
1 hard-boiled egg, chopped

For dressing:
1 Tbsp olive oil
Salt and pepper to taste
½ lemon,squeezed

Directions:

1. Place all the vegetables in a salad bowl.
2. Crumble the feta and sprinkle it, along with the roasted pumpkin seeds and egg, on top of the salad.
3. In a small bowl, pour the olive oil, add lemon juice, then add salt and pepper, and whisk together. Drizzle this dressing on top of the salad.
4. Toss gently before serving.

(Calories 45 | Total Fats 3g | Net Carbs: 3g | Protein 1g)

Bacon, Lettuce, Tomato Salad

(Total Time: 15 MIN| **Serve:** 4)

Ingredients:

1 cup of lettuce
1 spring onion
1 tomato
¼ cup toasted pumpkin seeds
Grated boiled egg
Sliced avocado
4 rashers of crispy bacon (crumbled)

For dressing:

1 Tbsp apple cider vinegar
1 tsp lemon juice
½ a finely crushed clove of garlic
1 Tbsp olive oil and some finely crushed fresh ginger (optional)

Directions:

1. In a large bowl combine salad ingredients
2. This can all be done at home and taken to work.
3. For dressing: In a separate container, mix dressing ingredients.
4. Allow the dressing to sit for a few hours.
5. Pour the dressing over the salad when you are ready to eat.

(Calories 288 | Total Fats 26g | Net Carbs: 7.4g | Protein 9.9g)

Broccoli Salad

(Total Time: 10 MIN| Serve: 4)

Ingredients:

1 cup broccoli
2 medium celery stalks
1/2 cup mushroom pieces (fried)
1/4 cup Cherry tomatoes
1 tbsp olive oil
2 cups Lettuce
1 Tbsp balsamic vinegar
½ cup pumpkin seeds, roasted dry in a pan

Directions:

1. Place all ingredients into a bowl, mix and enjoy.

(Calories 143 | Total Fats 11.6g | Net Carbs: 6.8g | Protein 5.5g)

Bacon with Cheesy Cauliflower Mash

(Total Time: 30 MIN| Serve: 3)

Ingredients:

4 cups cauliflower florets, chopped

3 Tbsp heavy cream

¼ tsp garlic powder

Salt and pepper to taste

4 bacon strips, cooked and chopped

1 cup cheddar cheese, shredded

Directions:

1. In an oven-safe bowl, mix the chopped cauliflower florets, heavy cream, butter, and season with the garlic powder, salt, and pepper.
2. Place the bowl in the microwave and cook on high for 20 minutes, or until the cauliflower is soft.
3. Pour the cooked cauliflower into a food processor and add the bacon and cheddar cheese.
4. Pulse until you achieve a smooth consistency.
5. Serve with a dab on of butter on top.

(Calories 590| Total Fats 51g | Net Carbs: 6g | Protein 22g)

Creamed Spinach

(Total Time: 15 MIN| Serve: 1)

Ingredients:

2 cup spinach
½ small onion, chopped
¼ cups water
1/2 stock cube
1 clove of garlic, chopped
¼ cups heavy cream
2 Tbsp butter
Salt and pepper to taste

Directions:

1. Place spinach and onion to a pan with water and heat over the medium-highheat.
2. Add the stock cube and garlic and allow to steam for 8-10 minutes, or until all the water has evaporated and the spinach is very soft.
3. Pour in the heavy cream and butter and then season with salt and pepper, cooking until it thickens.
4. Using a hand-held blender, blitz the spinach until fairly smooth.
5. Serve while hot.

(Calories 200 | Total Fats 23g | Net Carbs: 3g | Protein 7g)

Cheesy Zoodles with Fresh Basil

(Total Time: 15 MIN| Serve: 3)

Ingredients:

2 cups zucchini noodles (zoodles)
2 Tbsp fresh chopped basil
1/4 cup pecorino Romano cheese, shaved
1/4 cup grana padano cheese, grated
3 Tbsp salted butter
3 cloves mashed garlic
1 tsp red pepper flakes
1 Tbsp chopped red pepper
1 Tbsp coconut oil
Salt and fresh cracked pepper to taste

Directions:

1. In a frying pan over medium heat, melt butter and coconut oil. Add in garlic, chopped red pepper, and red pepper flakes. Sauté for 1 minute only.
2. Add in the zoodles and let cook for 1-2 minutes. Turn off heat and toss with fresh basil. Toss lightly.
3. Add in pecorino Romano cheese and toss.
4. Finally, sprinkle on top with grated grana padano cheese.
5. Serve immediately.

(Calories 314 | Total Fats 26g | Net Carbs: 6.1g | Protein 15g)

Veggie Burger Patties

(Total Time: 20 MIN| Serve: 4)

Ingredients:

2 cups Brussels sprouts
3 organic eggs
1 cup parmesan cheese, grated
1 ½ cups goat cheese
½ cup green onion, chopped
1/3 cup almond flour
1 cup parmesan cheese
Salt and pepper to taste

Directions:

1. Thoroughly wash the Brussels sprouts and place in the food processor to shred into pieces.
2. Transfer the Brussels sprouts to a bowl and add the parmesan cheese, goats cheese, green onion and almond flour into the bowl. Season with salt and pepper.
3. In another bowl, whisk the eggs and then pour over the Brussels sprouts mixture. Combine well using your hands.
4. Create burger patties, about 4 oz. each and then fry in a greased cast iron skillet for about 2 minutes on each side, or until crispy.

(Calories 182 | Total Fats 11g | Net Carbs: 7g | Protein 14g)

Mascarpone Zucchini Rolls

(Total Time: 15 MIN| Serve: 2)

Ingredients:

1 large zucchini cut thin using a mandolin
6 oz. mascarpone cheese
1 tsp dill, dried
1 tsp mint, dried
Salt and pepper to taste
1 Tbsp melted butter

Directions:

1. Brush the zucchini slices with the melted butter and season with salt and pepper
2. Heat your grill and place the zucchini. Cook for 2 minutes on each side.
3. In a bowl, combine the mascarpone, dill, and mint and whisk well.
4. Equally, scoop the mascarpone mixture on top of the grilled zucchini and spread.
5. Roll the zucchini and secure with toothpicks.
6. Serve and consume immediately.

(Calories 186| Total Fats 14g | Net Carbs: 3g | Protein 13g)

Tasty Cauliflower Rice

(Total Time: 25 MIN| Serve: 2)

Ingredients:

4 cups cauliflower florets
1 small onion, diced
2 cloves of garlic, minced
1 ½ tsp garlic powder
1½ tsp cumin
1 ½ tsp chili powder
Salt to taste
1 tbsp ghee
1 cup cheddar cheese, shredded
4 Tbsp sour cream

Directions:

1. Heat the ghee in a skillet over medium fire.
2. Add the onions into the hot pan and sauté for 3 minutes.
3. While waiting for the onions to cook, place the cauliflower florets in a food processor and pulse until they are chopped.
4. Throw in the garlic into the pan and sauté for another half a minute.
5. Add the chopped cauliflower to the pan, along with the garlic powder, cumin, chili powder, and season with salt.
6. Cook the cauliflower for 12-15 minutes or until tender.
7. Turn off the heat and transfer the cauliflower rice into serving bowls.
8. Top with the shredded cheese and sour cream while hot.

(Calories 618| Total Fats 48g | Net Carbs: 17g | Protein 27g)

Roquefort Spinach, Zoodles and Bacon Salad

(Total Time: 5 MIN| Serve: 5)

Ingredients:

4 cups of zucchini noodles
1 cup fresh broccoli
1/2 cup crumbled bacon
1 cup fresh spinach
1/3 cup Roquefort, bleu cheese, crumbled
1/3 cup bleu cheese dressing
Fresh cracked pepper (to taste)

Directions:

1. In a deep bowl, add all the ingredients together and toss lightly with a wooden spoon.
2. Serve and enjoy.

(Calories 81.2 | Total Fats 3.1g | Net Carbs: 9.5g | Protein 6g)

Spinach and Cheese Stuffed Mushrooms

(Total Time: 20 MIN| Serve: 6)

Ingredients:

12 large mushroom caps with stems
1 cream cheese
1 cup cooked, chopped spinach
1 Tbsp garlic, minced
1 tsp red pepper flakes
2 scallions, finely chopped
1 tsp salt
1 tsp fresh cracked pepper
3 tsp extra virgin olive oil
2 Tbsp almond, ground
2 Tbsp parmesan cheese
1 tsp granulated garlic
1 Tbsp fresh flat leaf parsley, finely chopped

Directions:

1. Preheat oven to 400 F.
2. First, remove the mushroom stems and chop the stems into small pieces.
3. Heat 2 tsp of olive oil in a frying pan and sauté mushroom stems for about 5 minutes.
4. In a small bowl, mix cooked mushroom stems, cream cheese, chopped spinach, scallions, minced garlic, red pepper flakes, salt, and pepper.
5. Then mix parmesan cheese, ground almonds, granulated garlic and parsley in another small bowl.
6. Fill the inside of the mushroom tops with the mushroom mixture and cheese. Then add the ground almonds mixture over the top of each mushroom.
7. Sprinkle the last tsp of oil over the mushroom caps and add a little extra cheese on the top.
8. Bake in oven about 12 minutes.
9. Serve hot.

(Calories 138.32 | Total Fats 6.36g | Net Carbs: 6.98g | Protein 11.75g)

Baked Broccoli with Mushrooms and Parmesan

(Total Time: 35 MIN| Serve: 2)

Ingredients:

4 cups broccoli
2 cups mushrooms (chopped fine)
2 Tbsp minced garlic
1/2 tsp dried oregano
3 Tbsp grated parmesan
Salt and ground black pepper to taste

Directions:

1. Preheat oven to 300F. Line a baking sheet with parchment paper.
2. Wash and slice broccoli into florets.
3. In a bowl, toss broccoli and finely chopped mushrooms in olive oil.
4. Season with dried oregano, salt, and pepper to taste.
5. Spread all vegetables evenly over the prepared baking pan.
6. Bake for 20-25 minutes until the broccoli is browned.
7. When done, leave to cool 5 minutes, sprinkle with parmesan cheese and serve.

(Calories 138.26 | Total Fats 3.51g | Net Carbs: 4.86g | Protein 12.16g)

Ail Creamy Brussels sprouts

(Total Time: 15 MIN| Serve: 1)

Ingredients:

10 Brussels sprouts
4 cloves garlic
1/4 cup cream cheese
2 Tbsp extra virgin olive oil
1 tsp balsamic vinegar
Salt and pepper to taste

Directions:

1. Clean the Brussels sprouts discarding the first leaves and cut into julienne strips.
2. Peel and chop the garlic cloves.
3. In a frying pan, heat the olive oil and frythe Brussels sprouts and garlic,
4. When the garlic and sprouts are tender, turn off the heat and add the cheese. Let sit for a couple of minutes.
5. Transfer to plate and serve.

(Calories 223.26 | Total Fats 12.55g | Net Carbs: 5.21g | Protein 9.27g)

Spicy Cauliflower with Sujuk Sausages

(Total Time: 30 MIN| Serve: 4)

Ingredients:

4 cups frozen cauliflower

8 oz sujuk sausages sliced (or red pastrami)

1 green pepper, chopped

1 tsp Cajun seasoning

1/2 onion, chopped

2 Tbsp minced garlic

2 Tbsp olive oil

Directions:

1. In a frying pan, sauté onion in olive oil for 2-3 minutes.
2. Squeeze the liquid from chopped cauliflower and add it to the pan. Sauté the cauliflower with onion for 5-10 minutes.
3. Add in Cajun seasoning and mix. Add in chopped sujuk sausages or pastrami and green peppers.
4. Toss and cook until about 5 minutes. Transfer to the plates and serve.

(Calories 181 | Total Fats 10g | Net Carbs: 9g | Protein 14g)

Chapter 10: Desserts & Fat Bombs

All-stars Peanut-Butter Cookies

(Total Time: 1 HR 15 MIN| Serve: 18)

Ingredients:

2 cups peanut butter
1/4 cup erythritol
2 eggs
1 1/4 cups coconut flour
2 tsp baking soda
2 tsp peanut extract
1/2 tsp kosher salt

Directions:

1. Preheat oven to 345 F.
2. In a bowl beat the peanut butter, coconut flour and erythritol with an electric mixer (Medium speed) until fluffy. Reduce speed to Low and add in the eggs, baking soda, vanilla, and salt.
3. With your hands, make balls from the batter and place on parchment-lined baking pan. Bake 10 to 15 minutes.
4. When ready, cool slightly and then move from the stove to cool completely Before serving.

(Calories 182.5 | Total Fats 14.67g | Net Carbs: 8.65g | Protein 7g)

Almond Chocolate Brownies

(Total Time: 35 MIN| Serve: 16)

Ingredients:

3 eggs
4 oz dark chocolate, unsweetened
1/2 cup coconut oil
1 cup almond flour
1 cup walnuts, chopped
2 Tbsp cocoa, unsweetened
1 tsp vanilla essence
2 cups granulated sweetener stevia or erythritol
1 tsp baking soda
Pinch of salt

Directions:

1. Preheat the oven to 350 F.
2. In a container, add almond flour, sweetener, cocoa, salt and baking soda. With an electric mixer, blend the ingredients on the lowest setting until combined well.
3. Melt the chocolate and the coconut oil together. Stir thoroughly.
4. Add eggs and vanilla essence to the flour and mix on a medium speed, until a thick batter is formed.
5. Add the butter/chocolate mix to the batter, continuing on medium speed until an even texture is formed.
6. Line a slice tin or square baking tin with wax paper.
7. Fold in chopped walnut then turn the batter into your slice tin.
8. Bake for 25 minutes.
9. Cut into 16 Brownies and serve.

(Calories 207.88 | Total Fats 20.72g | Net Carbs: 5.38g | Protein 5.14g)

Almond Chocolate Cookies

(Total Time: 25 MIN| Serve: 12)

Ingredients:

2 cups almond meal
1 1/2 tsp almond extract
4 Tbsp cocoa powder
5 Tbsp coconut oil, melted
2 Tbsp almond milk
4 Tbsp agave nectar
2 tsp vanilla extract
1/8 tsp baking soda
1/8 tsp salt

Directions:

1. Preheat oven to 340F degrees.
2. In a deep bowl mix salt, cocoa powder, almond meal and baking soda.
3. In a separate bowl, whisk together melted coconut oil, almond milk, almond and vanilla extract and maple syrup. Merge the almond meal mixture with almond milk mixture and mix well.
4. In a greased baking pan, pour the batter evenly. Bake for 10-15 minutes. 5. Once ready let cool on a wire rack, slice and serve.

(Calories 79.32 | Total Fats 5.94g | Net Carbs: 7.2g | Protein 0.46g)

Carrot Muffins

(Total Time: 50 MIN| Serve: 12)

Ingredients:

2 eggs

2 cups shredded carrots

1/4 cup coconut flour

1/2 cup coconut oil

1 tsp vanilla extract

1/4 cup erythritol

2 tsp ground cinnamon

1 tsp baking powder

Directions:

1. Preheat oven to 350F. Prepare 12 muffin tins.
2. In your food processor, add in carrots, eggs, coconut oil, erythritol, and vanilla. Blend together until combined.
3. In a separate bowl, mix together coconut flour, cinnamon, and baking powder.
4. Pour the carrot mixture into the dry ingredients and mix until completely combined.
5. Pour carrot mixture into the muffin tin and bake for about 30-35 minutes.
6. Remove from the oven, and let cool for at least 30 minutes before serving.

(Calories 127.55 | Total Fats 10.4g | Net Carbs: 8.81g | Protein 1.53g)

Coconut Jelly Cake

(Total Time: 30 MIN| **Serve:** 18)

Ingredients:

1 cup coconut flour

1/2 cup butter, softened

2 Tbsp raspberry jelly

1/2 cup coconut sugar

3 cups desiccated coconut

1 egg

2/3 cup coconut milk

1 cup boiling water

1 cup cold water

1/2 cup double thick cream

Directions:

1. Preheat oven to 360F. Grease a patty pan.
2. In a bowl beat coconut sugar and butter until light.
3. Add in egg and beat until well combined. Gently fold in half the coconut flour and half the milk. Repeat with remaining flour and milk.
4. Spoon mixture into patty pan. Bake for 15 to 20 minutes. Once ready, let cool cakes on a wire rack.
5. Stir boiling water and jelly together in a bowl until dissolved.
6. Stir in cold water and place in refrigerator for 1 hour.
7. Place coconut into a large bowl.
8. Cut each cake into the half.
9. Stick halves back together using 1 tsp of cream.
10. Using a spoon, lower cakes, 1 cake at a time, into jelly.
11. Toss cakes in coconut.
12. When ready, place onto a lined tray and refrigerate for 1 hour.

(Calories 146.51 | Total Fats 14.31g | Net Carbs: 4.21g | Protein 1.83g)

Cottage Pumpkin Pie Ice Cream

(Total Time: 15 MIN| Serve: 6)

Ingredients:

1/2 cup toasted pecans, chopped
3 egg yolks
2 Tbsp butter, salted
2 cups coconut milk
1/2 cup pumpkin puree
1 tsp pumpkin spice
1/2 cup cottage cheese
1/2 tsp chia seeds
1/3 cup erythritol
20 drops liquid Nutria

Directions:

1. Place all ingredients into a container of your immersion blender. Blend all of the ingredients together into a smooth mixture.
2. Add mixture to your ice cream machine.
3. Churn the ice cream using ice cream maker manufacturer's instructions.
4. Serve in a chilled bowl and enjoy.

(Calories 233.69 | Total Fats 21.74g | Net Carbs: 6.87g | Protein 5.49g)

Divine Keto Chocolate Biscotti

(Total Time: 25 MIN| Serve: 8)

Ingredients:

1 egg
2 cups whole almonds
2 Tbsp flax seeds
1 cup shredded coconut, unsweetened
1 cup coconut oil
1 cup cacao powder
1/4 cup xylitol or stevia sweetener
1 tsp salt
1 tsp baking soda

Directions:

1. Preheat oven to 350 F.
2. In a food processor, blend the almonds with the flax seeds.
3. Add in the rest of ingredients and mix well.
4. Place the dough on a piece of aluminum foil to shape into eight biscotti-shaped slices.
5. Bake in preheated oven for 12 minutes.
6. Let cool and serve.

(Calories 276.56 | Total Fats 25.44g | Net Carbs: 9.19g | Protein 8.24g)

Halloween Pumpkin Ice Cream

(Total Time: 15 MIN| Serve: 6)

Ingredients:

1 cup almond milk (unsweetened)
1 cup coconut milk
1 cup pumpkin puree
2 1/2 tsp ground cinnamon
1 tsp pure vanilla extract
1/2 tsp ground ginger
1/2 tsp nutmeg
1/8 tsp sea salt

Thickener:
1/2 tsp guar gum or 1 Tbsp gelatin dissolved in 1/4 cup boiling water

Directions:

1. Put the coconut milk in a blender and purée until smooth.
2. Freeze for about an hour or refrigerate until cold.
3. Add the almond milk, pumpkin puree, vanilla, cinnamon, ginger, nutmeg, and salt, plus a thickener. Purée until smooth.
4. Pour into the ice cream machine or blender and churn well.
5. Serve in chilled glasses.

(Calories 118.25 | Total Fats 11.3g | Net Carbs: 4.73g | Protein 1.35g)

Homemade Nut Bars

(Total Time: 15 MIN| Serve: 10)

Ingredients:

1 cup almonds
1/2 cup hazelnuts, chopped
1 cup peanuts
1 cup shredded coconut
1 cup almond butter
1 cup liquid erythritol
1 cup coconut oil, freshly melted and still warm

Directions:

1. In a food processor, place all nuts and chop for 1-2 minutes.
2. Add in grated coconut, almond butter, erythritol and coconut oil. Process it for about 1 minute.
3. Cover a square bowl with parchment paper and place the mixture on top.
4. Flatten the mixture with a spatula. Place the bowl in the freezer for 4-5 hours.
5. Remove batter from the freezer, cut and serve.

(Calories 193.62 | Total Fats 18.2g | Net Carbs: 6.64g | Protein 3.83g)

Chia Seed Cream

(Total Time: 12 HR| **Serve:** 4)

Ingredients:

1/4 cup Chia seeds

1 cup heavy whipping cream

1 cup coconut milk

2 Tbsp cocoa powder

Pure vanilla extract

1/4 cup erythritol sweetener

Directions:

1. In a bowl, mix the chia seeds and add the coconut milk, until it combines well.
2. Add the erythritol and whisk some more. Divide the mixture into two portions.
3. Add cocoa to one-half and mixed it nicely.
4. Pour chia seed mixture into bowls or glasses. Keep covered in the refrigerator for 12 hours.
5. Before serving, beat the heavy whipping cream and pour over the chia seeds cream. Enjoy!

(Calories 341.31 | Total Fats 35.41g | Net Carbs: 7.35g | Protein 2.99g)

Hemp and Chia Seeds Cream

(Total Time: 20 MIN| **Serve:** 3)

Ingredients:

1 ¼ cup coconut milk

2 Tbsp hemp powder

2 sheets of unflavored gelatin

3 Tbsp chia seeds

Directions:

1. In a saucepan over low heat, add the coconut milk and dissolve the hemp powder.
2. Cut the gelatin into pieces and add it to the milk. Stir until dissolved completely.
3. Add chia seeds and stir occasionally until mixture thickens, about 15 minutes.
4. Pour the mixture into individual containers and allow to cool, before putting them in the refrigerator for at least 2 hours before serving. Enjoy!

(Calories 202.43 | Total Fats 160.45g | Net Carbs: 8.12g | Protein 2.59g)

Chocolate Brownies

(Total Time: 35 MIN| Serve: 10)

Ingredients:

2 eggs
1 1/2 cups almond flour
1/4 cup coconut oil
1/2 cup cocoa powder, unsweetened
1 Tbsp Metamucil Fiber Powder
1/3 cup Natvia (or some other natural sweetener)l
1/4 cup maple syrup
1 tsp baking powder
1/2 tsp salt

Directions:

1. Preheat oven to 350 F.
2. In a bowl, add in all wet ingredients and 2 Eggs. Beat the wet ingredients together using a hand mixer until a consistent mixture is formed.
3. In a separate bowl, combine all dry ingredients. Mix the dry ingredients well.
4. Pour the wet ingredients slowly into the dry ingredients, mixing with a hand mixer as you pour.
5. Pour the batter into baking pan. Bake the brownies for 20 minutes.
6. When ready, let the brownies cool. Slice brownies into slices and serve.

(Calories 157.81 | Total Fats 13.4g | Net Carbs: 8.7g | Protein 5.4g)

Chocolate Pecan Bites

(Total Time: 3 HR| Serve: 12)

Ingredients:

2 oz 100% dark chocolate

2.5 oz pecan halves

Cinnamon

Nutmeg

Directions:

1. Preheat oven to 350 F.
2. Place the pecan halves on a parchment paper and bake in the oven for 6-7 minutes. When ready, let cool and set aside.
3. Melt the dark chocolate.
4. Dip each pecan half in the melted dark chocolate and place back on the parchment paper.
5. Sprinkle cinnamon and nutmeg on top of the chocolate covered pecans.
6. Before serving, place in refrigerator for 2-3 hours.

(Calories 52.13 | Total Fats 4.96g | Net Carbs: 2.32g | Protein 0.64g)

Creamy Chocolate Mousse

(Total Time: 15 MIN| Serve: 4)

Ingredients:

1/4 cup of heavy cream

1 1/4 cup coconut cream

2 Tbsp of cocoa powder

3 Tbsp of erythritol (or stevia)

1 Tbsp pure vanilla essence

Shredded coconut, unsweetened

Directions:

1. Add coconut cream and heavy cream into a bowl & combine, using a hand mixer on low speed.
2. Add the remaining ingredients and mix on low speed for 2-3 minutes, until the mixture is thick.
3. Serve in individual ramekins, sprinkled with unsweetened shredded coconut.

(Calories 305.19 | Total Fats 31.91g | Net Carbs: 6.97g | Protein 3.56g)

Hazelnut Chocolate Cream

(Total Time: 5 MIN| Serve: 4)

Ingredients:

1 cup hazelnut halves

4 Tbsp unsweetened cocoa powder

1 tsp pure vanilla extract

2 Tbsp coconut oil

4 Tbsp granulated stevia (or sweetener of choice)

Directions:

1. Place all the ingredients in your blender. Blend until smooth well.
2. Place in the fridge for 1 hour. Serve and enjoy!

(Calories 302.88 | Total Fats 29.65g | Net Carbs: 9.5g | Protein 6.39g)

Lemon Coconut Pearls

(Total Time: 15 MIN| Serve: 4)

Ingredients:

3 packages of True Lemon (Crystallized Citrus for Water)

1/4 cup shredded coconut, unsweetened

1 cup cream cheese

1/4 cup granulated stevia

Directions:

1. In a bowl, combine cream cheese, lemon, and stevia. Blend well until incorporated.
2. Once the mixture is well combined, put it back in the fridge to harden up a bit.
3. Roll into 16 balls and dip each ball into shredded coconut.
4. Refrigerate for several hours. Serve.

(Calories 216.06 | Total Fats 21.53g | Net Carbs: 3.12g | Protein 3.61g)

Instant Coffee Ice Cream

(Total Time: 20 MIN| **Serve:** 2)

Ingredients:

1 Tbsp instant coffee
2 Tbsp cocoa powder
1 cup coconut milk
1/4 cup heavy cream
1/4 tsp flax seeds
2 Tbsp erythritol
15 drops liquid Nutria

Directions:

1. Add all ingredients except the flax seeds into a container of your immersion blender.
2. Blend well until all ingredients are incorporated well.
3. Slowly add in flax seeds, until a slightly thicker mixture is formed.
4. Add the mass to your ice cream machine and follow manufacturer's instructions.
5. Serve and enjoy!

(Calories 286.99 | Total Fats 29.21g | Net Carbs: 9.39g | Protein 3.18g)

Jam "Eye" Cookies

(Total Time: 36 MIN| Serve: 16)

Ingredients:

2 eggs
1 cup almond flour
2 Tbsp coconut flour
2 Tbsp sugar-free jam per taste
1/2 cup natural sweetener
4 tbsp coconut oil
1/2 tsp pure vanilla extract
1/2 tsp almond extract
1 tbsp shredded coconut
1/2 tsp baking powder
1/4 tsp cinnamon
1/2 tsp salt

Directions:

1. Preheat your oven to 350 F. In a big bowl, combine all your dry ingredients and whisk.
2. Add in your wet ingredients and combine well, using a hand mixer or a whisk.
3. Use your hands for making the patties and place the cookies on a parchment paper-lined baking sheet. Using your finger, make an indent in the middle of each cookie.
4. Bake for about 16 minutes, or until the cookies turn golden.
5. Once ready, let the cookies cool on a wire rack and fill each indent with sugar-free jam.
6. Before serving, sprinkle some shredded coconut on top of each cookie. Enjoy!

(Calories 95.1 | Total Fats 8.61g | Net Carbs: 2.79g | Protein 2.71g)

Lime & Vanilla Cheesecake

(Total Time: 2 HR 5 MIN| Serve: 2)

Ingredients:

1/4 cup cream cheese, softened
2 Tbsp heavy cream
1 tsp lime juice
1 egg
1 tsp pure vanilla extract
2-4 Tbsp erythritol or stevia

Directions:

1. In a microwave-safe bowl, combine all ingredients. Place in a microwave and cook on HIGH for 90 seconds.
2. Every 30 seconds, stir to combine the ingredients well.
3. Transfer mixture to a bowl and refrigerate for at least 2 hours.
4. Before serving, top with whipped cream or coconut powder.

(Calories 140.42 | Total Fats 13.04g | Net Carbs: 1.38g | Protein 4.34g)

Strawberry Pudding

(Total Time: 35 MIN| Serve: 3)

Ingredients:

4 egg yolks
2 Tbsp butter
1/4 cup coconut flour
2 Tbsp heavy cream
1/4 cup strawberries
1/4 tsp baking powder
2 Tbsp coconut oil
2 tsp lemon juice
Zest 1 lemon
2 Tbsp erythritol
10 drops liquid stevia

Directions:

1. Preheat oven to 350 F.
2. In a bowl, beat the egg yolks with electric mixer until they're pale in color. Add in erythritol and 10 drops liquid stevia. Beat again until fully combined.
3. Add in heavy cream, lemon juice, and the zest of 1 lemon. Add the coconut and butter. Beat well until no lumps are found.
4. Sift the dry ingredients over the wet ingredients, and then mix well on a slow speed.
5. Distribute the strawberries evenly in the batter by pushing them into the top of the batter.
6. Bake for 20-25 minutes. Once finished, let cool for 5 minutes and serve.

(Calories 258.65 | Total Fats 23.46g | Net Carbs: 9.3g | Protein 3.98g)

Kiwi Fiend Ice Cream

(Total Time: 8 HR 15 MIN| Serve: 6)

Ingredients:

3 egg yolks
1 1/2 cup kiwi, pureed
1 cup heavy cream
1/3 cup erythritol
1/2 tsp pure vanilla extract
1/8 tsp chia seeds

Directions:

1. In a saucepan, heat up the heavy cream. Add erythritol and simmer until the erythritol has dissolved.
2. Beat 3 egg yolks in a medium sized mixing bowl with an electric mixer. Add in hot cream mixture, 1 tsp at a time to the eggs, while beating. Add in some pure vanilla extract and mix. Add in 1/8 tsp. of chia seeds.
3. Once the ingredients are combined, put your bowl into the freezer and let it chill for 1-2 hours, stirring twice.
4. In a meanwhile, puree the kiwi for no more than 1-2 seconds. When the ice cream is getting a bit thicker, about 1 hour in, add the kiwi mixture to the cream and mix well.
5. Let the kiwi ice cream to chill at least 6-8 hours. Serve in chilled glasses.

(Calories 192.47 | Total Fats 17.2g | Net Carbs: 8.13g | Protein 2.69g)

Minty Avocado Lime Sorbet

(Total Time: 3 HR 15 MIN| Serve: 6)

Ingredients:

1 cup coconut milk

2 avocados, sliced vertically into 5 pieces

1/4 mint leaves, chopped

1/4 cup powdered erythritol

2 limes, juiced

1/4 tsp liquid stevia

Directions:

1. Place avocado pieces on foil and squeeze the ½ lime juice over the top.
2. Place avocado in the freezer for at least 3 hours.
3. Using a spice grinder, powder erythritol.
4. In a pan, bring coconut milk to a boil.
5. Zest the 2 limes while coconut milk is heating up. Add lime zest and continue to let the milk reduce in volume.
6. Remove and place the coconut milk into a container and store in the freezer.
7. Chop mint leaves. Remove avocados from the freezer.
8. Add avocado, mint leaves, and juice from lime into the food processor. Pulse until a chunky consistency is achieved.
9. Pour coconut milk mixture over the avocados in the food processor. Add liquid stevia to this.
10. Pulse mixture together about 2-3 minutes.
11. Return to freezer to freeze, or serve immediately!

(Calories 184.18 | Total Fats 17.26g | Net Carbs: 9.65g | Protein 1.95g)

Morning Zephyr Cake

(Total Time: 40 MIN| Serve: 8)

Ingredients:

3 Tbsp coconut oil

2 Tbsp ground flax seeds

8 Tbsp almonds, ground

1 cup Greek yogurt

1 Tbsp cocoa powder for dusting

1 cup heavy whipping cream

1 tsp baking powder

1 tsp baking soda

1 tsp pure vanilla essence

1 pinch pink salt

1 cup stevia or erythritol sweetener

Directions:

1. Pre-heat the oven to 350 F degrees.
2. In the blender, first add the ground almonds, ground flax seeds, and the baking powder and soda. Blend for a minute.
3. Add the salt, coconut oil and blend some more. Add the sweetener and blend for 2-3 minutes.
4. Add the Greek yogurt and blend for a minute or so, until a fine consistency is reached.
5. Take out the batter, place in a bowl and add the vanilla essence, and mix with a light hand.
6. Grease the baking dish and drop the batter in it.
7. Bake for 30 minutes. Let cool on a wire rack. Serve.

(Calories 199.84 | Total Fats 20.69g | Net Carbs: 3.22g | Protein 2.56g)

Peanut Butter Balls

(Total Time: 22 MIN| Serve: 16)

Ingredients:

2 eggs
2 1/2 cup of peanut butter
1/2 cup shredded coconut (unsweetened)
1/2 cup of xylitol
1 Tbsp of pure vanilla extract

Directions:

1. Preheat oven to 320 F.
2. Mix all ingredients together by hand.
3. After the ingredients are thoroughly mixed, roll into heaped Tbsp sized balls and press into a baking tray lined with baking paper.
4. Bake in preheated oven for 12 minutes.
5. When ready, let cool on a wire rack.
6. Serve and enjoy.

(Calories 254.83 | Total Fats 21.75g | Net Carbs: 8.31g | Protein 10.98g)

Pecan Flax Seed Blondies

(Total Time: 40 MIN| Serve: 16)

Ingredients:

3 eggs
2 1/4 cups pecans, roasted
3 Tbsp heavy cream
1 Tbsp salted caramel syrup
1/2 cup flax seeds, ground
1/4 cup butter, melted
1/4 cup erythritol, powdered
10 drops liquid stevia
1 tsp baking powder
1 pinch salt

Directions:

1. Preheat oven to 350F.
2. In a baking pan, roast pecans for 10 minutes.
3. Grind 1/2 cup flax seeds in a spice grinder. Place flax seed powder in a bowl. Grind erythritol in a spice grinder until powdered. Set in the same bowl as the flax seed meal.
4. Place 2/3 of roasted pecans in food processor and process until smooth nut butter is formed.
5. Add eggs, liquid stevia, salted caramel syrup, and a pinch of salt to the flax seed mixture. Mix well. Add pecan butter to the batter and mix again.
6. Crush the remaining roasted pecans into chunks.
7. Add crushed pecans and 1/4 cup melted butter into the batter.
8. Mix batter well and then add heavy cream and baking powder. Mix everything together well.
9. Place the batter into baking tray and bake for 20 minutes.
10. Let cool for about 10 minutes.
11. Cut into squares and serve.

(Calories 180.45 | Total Fats 18.23g | Net Carbs: 3.54g | Protein 3.07g)

Peppermint Chocolate Ice Cream

(Total Time: 35 MIN| Serve: 3)

Ingredients:

1/2 tsp peppermint extract
1 cup heavy cream
1 cup cheese cream
1 tsp pure vanilla extract
1 tsp liquid stevia extract
100% dark chocolate for topping

Directions:

1. Place ice cream bowl in the freezer.
2. In a metal bowl, add all ingredients, except chocolate, and whisk well.
3. Put back in the freezer for 5 minutes.
4. Set up ice cream maker and add liquid.
5. Before serving, top the ice cream with chocolate shavings. Serve.

(Calories 286.66 | Total Fats 29.96g | Net Carbs: 2.7g | Protein 2.6g)

Puff-up Coconut Waffles

(Total Time: 20 MIN| Serve: 8)

Ingredients:

1 cup coconut flour
1/2 cup heavy (whipping) cream
5 eggs
1/4 tsp pink salt
1/4 tsp baking soda
1/4 cup coconut milk
2 tsp yacon syrup
2 Tbsp coconut oil (melted)

Directions:

1. In a large bowl, add the eggs and beat with an electric hand mixer for 30 seconds.
2. Add the heavy (whipping) cream and coconut oil into the eggs while you are still mixing. Add the coconut milk, coconut flour, pink salt and baking soda. Mix with the hand mixer for 45 seconds on low speed. Set aside.
3. Heat up your waffle maker well and make the waffles according to your manufacturer's specifications.
4. Serve hot.

(Calories 169.21 | Total Fats 12.6g | Net Carbs: 9.97g | Protein 4.39g)

Raspberry Chocolate Cream

(Total Time: 15 MIN| Serve: 4)

Ingredients:

1/2 cup 100% dark chocolate, chopped
1/4 cup of heavy cream
1/2 cup cream cheese, softened
2 Tbsp sugar-free raspberry syrup
1/4 cup erythritol

Directions:

1. In a double boiler, melt chopped chocolate and the cream cheese. Add the erythritol sweetener and continue to stir. Remove from heat, let cool and set aside.
2. When the cream has cooled, add in heavy cream and raspberry syrup and stir well.
3. Pour cream in a bowls or glasses and serve. Keep refrigerated.

(Calories 157.67 | Total Fats 13.51g | Net Carbs: 7.47g | Protein 1.95g)

Raw Cacao Hazelnut Cookies

(Total Time: 6 HR| Serve: 24)

Ingredients:

2 cups almond flour
1 cup chopped hazelnuts
1/2 cup cacao powder
1/2 cup ground flax
3 Tbsp coconut oil (melted)
1/3 cup water
1/3 cup erythritol
1/4 tsp liquid stevia

Directions:

1. In a bowl, mix flax and almond flour, cacao powder.
2. Stir in oil, water, erythritol and stevia, plus vanilla. When it is well combined, stir in chopped hazelnuts.
3. Form into balls, press flat with palms and place on dehydrator screens.
4. Dehydrate one hour at 145, then reduce to 116 and dehydrate for at least five hours.
5. Serve and enjoy.

(Calories 181.12 | Total Fats 15.69g | Net Carbs: 8.75g | Protein 4.46g)

Sinless Pumpkin Cheesecake Muffins

(Total Time: 15 MIN| Serve: 6)

Ingredients:

1/2 cup pureed pumpkin
1 tsp pumpkin pie spice
1/2 cup pecans, finely ground
1/2 cup cream cheese
1 Tbsp coconut oil
1/2 tsp pure vanilla extract
1/4 tsp pure yacon syrup or erythritol

Directions:

1. Prepare a muffin tin with liners.
2. Place a few ground pecans into every muffin tin and make a thin crust.
3. In a bowl, blend sweetener, spices, vanilla, coconut and the pumpkin puree. Add in the cream cheese and beat until the mixture is well combined.
4. Scoop about two Tbsp of filling mixture on top of each crust, and smooth the edges.
5. Pop in the freezer for about 45 minutes.
6. Remove from the muffin tin and let sit for 10 minutes. Serve.

(Calories 157.34 | Total Fats 15.52g | Net Carbs: 3.94g | Protein 2.22g)

Sour Hazelnuts Biscuits with Arrowroot Tea

(Total Time: 50 MIN| Serve: 12)

Ingredients:

1 egg
1/2 cup hazelnuts
3 Tbsp of coconut oil
2 cups almond flour
2 Tbsp of arrowroot tea
2 tsp ginger
1 Tbsp cocoa powder
1/2 cup grapefruit juice
1 orange peel from a half orange
1/2 tsp baking soda
1 pinch of salt

Directions:

1. Preheat oven to 360 F.
2. Make arrowroot tea and let it cool.
3. In a food processor, blend the hazelnuts. Add the remaining ingredients and continue blending until mixed well. With your hands, form cookies with the batter.
4. Put the cookies on baking parchment paper, and bake for 30-35 minutes. When ready, remove the tray from the oven and let cool.
5. Serve warm or cold.

(Calories 224.08 | Total Fats 20.17g | Net Carbs: 8.06g | Protein 6.36g)

Tartar Keto Cookies

(Total Time: 35 MIN| Serve: 8)

Ingredients:

3 eggs
1/8 tsp cream of tartar
1/3 cup cream cheese
1/8 tsp salt
Some oil for greasing

Directions:

1. Preheat oven to 300 F.
2. Line the cookie sheet with parchment paper and grease with some oil.
3. Separate eggs from the egg yolks. Set both in different mixing bowls.
4. With an electric hand mixer, start beating the egg whites until super bubbly. Add in cream of tartar and beat until stiff peaks form.
5. In the egg yolk bowl, add in cream cheese and some salt. Beat until the egg yolks are pale yellow.
6. Fold the egg whites into the cream cheese mixture using a metal spoon. Stir well.
7. Make cookies and place on the cookie sheet.
8. Bake for about 30-40 minutes. When ready, let them cool on a wire rack and serve.

(Calories 59.99 | Total Fats 5.09g | Net Carbs: 0.56g | Protein 2.93g)

Wild Strawberries Ice Cream

(Total Time: 5 MIN| Serve: 4)

Ingredients:

1/2 cup wild strawberries

1/3 cup cream cheese

1 cup heavy cream

1 Tbsp lemon juice

1 tsp pure vanilla extract

1/3 cup of your favorite sweetener

Ice cubes

Directions:

1. Place all ingredients in a blender. Blend until all ingredients are incorporated well.
2. Refrigerate for 2-3 hour before serving.

(Calories 176.43 | Total Fats 17.69g | Net Carbs: 3.37g | Protein 1.9g)

Mini Lemon Cheesecakes

(Total Time: 5 MIN| Serve: 6)

Ingredients:

1 tbsp lemon zest, grated

1 tsp lemon juice

½ tsp stevia powder (or Truvia)

1/4 cup coconut oil, softened

4 Tbsp unsalted butter, softened

4 ounces cream cheese (heavy cream)

Directions:

1. Blend all ingredients together with a hand mixer or blender, until smooth and creamy.
2. Prepare a cupcake or muffin tin with 6 paper liners.
3. Pour mixture into prepared tin and place in freezer for 2-3 hours or until firm.
4. Sprinkle cups with additional lemon zest. Or try using chopped nuts or shredded, unsweetened coconut.

(Calories 213 | Total Fats 23g | Net Carbs: 0.7g | Protein 1.5g)

Chocolate Layered Coconut Cups

(Total Time: 55 MIN| Serve: 10)

Ingredients:
Bottom Layer:
1/2 cup unsweetened, shredded coconut
3 Tbsp powdered sweeteners, such as Splenda or Truvia
1/2 cup coconut butter
1/2 cup coconut oil

Top Layer:
1 1/2 ounces cocoa butter
1-ounce unsweetened chocolate
1/4 cup cocoa powder
1/2 tsp vanilla extract
1/4 cup powdered sweetener such as Splenda or Truvia

Directions:

1. Prepare a mini-muffin pan with 20 mini paper liners.
2. For the bottom layer:
3. Combine coconut oil and coconut butter in a small saucepan over low heat.
4. Stir until smooth and melted, then add the shredded coconut and powdered sweetener, until well combined.
5. Divide the mixture among prepared mini muffin cups and place in the refrigerator for 30 minutes.
6. For the top layer:
7. Combine cocoa butter and unsweetened chocolate together in double boiler or a bowl set over a pan of simmering water. Stir until melted.
8. Stir in the powdered sweetener, then add the cocoa powder, and mix until smooth.
9. Remove from heat and stir in the vanilla extract.
10. Spoon chocolate mixture over coconut candies and let them set for 15 minutes.
11. Serve and enjoy.

(Calories 300| Total Fats 27g | Net Carbs: 14.5g | Protein 2g)

Pumpkin Pie Chocolate Cups

(Total Time: 45 MIN| Serve: 18)

Ingredients:

For the crust:

3.5 ounces extra dark chocolate - 85% cocoa solids or more

2 Tbsp coconut oil

For the pie:

½ cup coconut butter

¼ cup coconut oil

2 tsp pumpkin pie spice mix

½ cup unsweetened pumpkin puree

2 Tbsp healthy low-carb sweetener

Optional: 15-20 drops liquid stevia for added sweetness

Directions:

1. Place the chocolate and coconut oil in a double boiler or a glass bowl on top of a small saucepan filled with simmering water. Once completely melted, remove from the heat and set aside.
2. Prepare a mini muffin tin with 18 paper liners.
3. Fill each of the 18 mini muffin cups with 2 tsp of the chocolate mixture.
4. Place the chocolate in the refrigerator for 10 minutes.
5. Place the coconut butter, coconut oil, sweetener and pumpkin spice mix into a bowl and melt, just like you did the chocolate.
6. Add the pumpkin puree and mix until smooth and well combined.
7. Remove the muffin cups from the fridge and add a heaping tsp of the pumpkin & coconut mixture into every cup.
8. Place back in the refrigerator and let it sit for 30 minutes.
9. When done, keep refrigerated. Coconut oil and butter get very soft at room temperature.
10. Store in the refrigerator.
11. Serve and enjoy.

(Calories 92| Total Fats 9.1g | Net Carbs: 3.4g | Protein 0.7g)

Fudgy Cake

(Total Time: 3 HR 20 MIN| Serve: 10)

Ingredients:

1 1/2 cups almond flour

1/4 cup whey protein powder (chocolate, vanilla, and unflavored all work fine)

3/4 cup sugar substitute, such as Swerve or Truvia

2/3 cup cocoa powder

2 tsp baking powder

1/4 tsp sea salt

1/2 cup butter, melted

4 large eggs

3/4 cup almond or coconut milk, unsweetened

1 tsp vanilla extract

1/2 cup chopped dark chocolate, 85% cocoa or higher

Whipped cream topping (optional):

1/2 cup heavy whipping cream

2 Tbsp sugar substitute

Directions:

1. Grease the insert of a 6-quart slow cooker well with butter or coconut oil.
2. In a medium bowl, whisk together almond flour, sugar substitute, cocoa powder, whey protein powder, baking powder, and salt.
3. Stir in butter, eggs, almond milk and vanilla extract until well combined, then fold in the chopped dark chocolate.
4. Pour into the greased slow cooker and cook on low for 2.5 to 3 hours. It will be gooey and like a pudding cake at 2.5 hours and little more cake-like at 3 hours.
5. Turn slow cooker off and let cool for 20 to 30 minutes. Cut into pieces and serve warm.
6. Best when served with freshly whipped cream. To make this, mix the whipping cream and sugar substitute together with your stand mixer, or a hand mixer. Continue mixing until soft peaks form.

(Calories 313 | Total Fats 26g | Net Carbs: 14g | Protein 10g)

Easy Sticky Chocolate Fudge

(Total Time: 25 MIN| Serve: 12)

Ingredients:

1 cup coconut oil, softened
1/4 cup coconut milk (full fat, from a can)
1/4 cup cocoa powder
1 tsp vanilla extract
1/2 tsp sea salt
1-3 drops liquid stevia

Directions:

1. With a hand mixer or stand mixer, whip the softened coconut oil and coconut milk together until smooth and glossy. About 6 minutes on high.
2. Add the cocoa powder, vanilla extract, sea salt, and one drop of liquid stevia to the bowl and mix on low until combined. Increase speed once everything is combined and mix for one minute. Taste fudge and adjust sweetness by adding additional liquid stevia, if desired.
3. Prepare a 9"x4" loaf pan by lining it with parchment paper.
4. Pour fudge into loaf pan and place in freezer for about 15, until just set.
5. Remove fudge and cut into 1" x 1" pieces.
6. Store in an airtight container in the refrigerator.

(Calories 173 | Total Fats 19g | Net Carbs: 1.3g | Protein 0.4g)

Raspberry & Coconut Fat Bombs

(Total Time: 15 MIN| Serve: 12)

Ingredients:

1/2 cup coconut butter

1/2 cup coconut oil

1/2 cup freeze dried raspberries

1/2 cup unsweetened shredded coconut

1/4 powdered sugar substitute, such as Swerve or Truvia

Directions:

1. Line an 8"x8" pan with parchment paper.
2. In a food processor, coffee grinder or blender, pulse the dried raspberries into a fine powder.
3. In a saucepan over medium heat, combine the coconut butter, coconut oil, coconut, and sweetener. Stir until melted and well combined.
4. Remove pan from heat and stir in raspberry powder.
5. Pour mixture into the pan and refrigerate or freeze for several hours, or overnight.
6. Cut into 12 pieces and serve.

(Calories 189 | Total Fats 17.8g | Net Carbs: 7.9g | Protein 1.1g)

Strawberry Cheesecake Ice Cream Cups

(Total Time: 10 MIN| Serve: 12)

Ingredients:

1/2 strawberries, fresh or frozen, mashed well

3/4 cup cream cheese, softened

1/4 cup coconut oil, softened

10-15 drops liquid stevia

1 tsp vanilla extract

Directions:

1. Combine all ingredients in a medium-sized bowl and mix with a hand mixer, until smooth and creamy. (Can also be done in a food processor or high-speed blender.)
2. Spoon the mixture into mini muffin silicon molds or small candy molds. Place in the freezer for about 2 hours, or until set.
3. When done, unmold the fat bombs and place into a container. Keep in the freezer and enjoy anytime!

(Calories 91 | Total Fats 9.6g | Net Carbs: 0.5g | Protein 1.1g)

Buttery Pecan Delights

(Total Time: 15 MIN| Serve: 2)

Ingredients:

8 pecan halves

1 Tbsp unsalted butter, softened

2 ounces neufchâtel cheese

1 tsp orange zest, finely grated

Pinch of sea salt

Directions:

1. Toast the pecans at 350 degrees F for 5-10 minutes, check often to prevent burning.
2. Mix the butter, neufchâtel cheese, and orange zest until smooth and creamy.
3. Spread the butter mixture between the cooled pecan halves and sandwich together.
4. Sprinkle with sea salt and enjoy.

(Calories 129 | Total Fats 12.8g | Net Carbs: 1.2g | Protein 3g)

Peppermint Patties

(Total Time: 10 MIN| Serve: 12)

Ingredients:

¾ cup melted coconut butter

¼ cup finely shredded, unsweetened coconut

2 Tbsp cacao powder

3 Tbsp coconut oil, melted

½ tsp pure peppermint extract

Directions:

1. Mix together melted coconut butter, shredded coconut, 1 Tbsp of coconut oil and peppermint extract
2. Pour coconut butter mixture into mini muffin tins that have been lined with paper liners. Fill halfway.
3. Place in refrigerator and allow to harden for about 15 minutes.
4. Mix together 2 Tbsp coconut oil and cacao powder.
5. Remove muffin tin from the refrigerator and top each one with chocolate mixture.
6. Return to refrigerator until the chocolate has set.
7. When ready to eat, simply set the peppermint patty cups on the counter for about 5 minutes and unmold from muffin tin.

(Calories 137 | Total Fats 22.6g | Net Carbs: 4.4g | Protein 1.3g)

Chocolate Fudge

(Total Time: 20 MIN| Serve: 12)

Ingredients:

1 cup coconut oil, softened
1/4 cup coconut milk (full fat, from a can)
1/2 tsp sea salt
1-3 drops liquid stevia
1/4 cup cocoa powder
1 tsp vanilla extract

Directions:

1. With a hand mixer or stand mixer, whip the softened coconut oil and coconut milk together until smooth and glossy (about 6 minutes on high).
2. Add the cocoa powder, vanilla extract, sea salt, and one drop of liquid stevia to the bowl and mix on low until combined. Increase speed once everything is combined and mix for one minute. Taste fudge and adjust sweetness by adding additional liquid stevia, if desired.
3. Prepare a 9"x4" loaf pan by lining it with parchment paper.
4. Pour fudge into loaf pan and place in freezer for about 15, until just set.
5. Remove fudge and cut into 1" x 1" pieces.
6. Store in an airtight container in the refrigerator.

(Calories 173 | Total Fats 19.6g | Net Carbs: 1.3g | Protein 0.4g)

Cinna-Bun Balls

(Total Time: 15 MIN| **Serve:** 10)

Ingredients:

1 cup coconut butter
1 tsp vanilla extract
1 cup full-fat coconut milk (from a can)
1 cup unsweetened coconut shreds
1/2 tsp cinnamon
1/2 tsp nutmeg
1 tsp sugar substitute, such as Splenda

Directions:

1. Combine all ingredients, except the shredded coconut, together in double boiler or a bowl set over a pan of simmering water. Stir until everything is melted and combined.
2. Remove bowl from heat and place in the fridge until the mixture has firmed up and can be rolled into balls.
3. Form the mixture into 1" balls. A small cookie scoop is helpful for doing this.
4. Roll each ball in the shredded coconut, until well coated.
5. Serve and enjoy! Store in the fridge.

(Calories 280 | Total Fats 26.6g | Net Carbs: 9.9g | Protein 3g)

Vanilla Mousse Cups

(Total Time: 15 MIN| Serve: 6)

Ingredients:

8 ounces (1 block) cream cheese, softened
1/2 cup sugar substitute, such as Swerve or Truvia (stevia)
1 1/2 tsp vanilla extract
Dash of sea salt
1/2 cup heavy whipping cream

Directions:

1. Add the first four ingredients to a food processor or blender.
2. Blend until combined.
3. With blender running, slowly add the heavy cream.
4. Continue to blend until thickened, about 1-2 minutes. Consistency should be mousse-like.
5. Prepare a cupcake or muffin tin with 6 paper liners and portion the mixture into the cups.
6. Chill in the fridge until set and enjoy!

(Calories 170 | Total Fats 16.9g | Net Carbs: 1.6g | Protein 3.1g)

Rich & Creamy Fat Bomb Ice Cream

(Total Time: 20 MIN| Serve: 5)

Ingredients:

4 whole pastured eggs
4 yolks from pastured eggs
⅓ cup melted cocoa butter
⅓ cup melted coconut oil
15-20 drops liquid stevia
⅓ cup cocoa powder
¼ cup MCT oil
2 tsp pure vanilla extract
8-10 ice cubes

Directions:

1. Add all ingredients, but the ice cubes, into the jug of your high-speed blender. Blend on high for 2 minutes, until creamy.
2. While the blender is running, remove the top portion of the lid and drop in 1 ice cube at a time, allowing the blender to run about 10 seconds between each ice cube.
3. Once all of the ice has been added, pour the cold mixture into a 9x5" loaf pan and place in the freezer. Set the timer for 30 minutes before taking out to stir. Repeat this process for 2-3 hours, until desired consistency is met.
4. Serve immediately. Top with chopped nuts or shaved dark chocolate, if desired.
5. Store covered in the freezer for up to a week.

(Calories 448 | Total Fats 48.1g | Net Carbs: 4.1g | Protein 7.6g)

English Toffee Treats

(Total Time: 10 MIN| **Serve:** 24)

Ingredients:

1 cup coconut oil
2 Tbsp butter
4 ounces cream cheese, softened
3/4 Tbsp cocoa powder
1/2 cup creamy, natural peanut butter
3 Tbsp Davinci Gourmet Sugar-Free English Toffee Syrup

Directions:

1. Combine all ingredients in a saucepan over medium heat.
2. Stir until everything is smooth, melted, and combined.
3. Pour mixture into small candy molds, or mini muffin tins lined with paper liners.
4. Freeze or refrigerate until set and enjoy!
5. Store in an airtight container in the fridge.

(Calories 125 | Total Fats 13.4g | Net Carbs: 1.1g | Protein 1.3g)

Fudgy Peanut Butter Squares

(Total Time: 10 MIN| Serve: 12)

Ingredients:

1 cup all natural creamy peanut butter
1 cup coconut oil
1/4 cup unsweetened vanilla almond milk
a pinch of coarse sea salt
1 tsp vanilla extract
2 tsp liquid stevia (optional)

Directions:

1. In a microwave-safe bowl, soften the peanut butter and coconut oil together. (About 1 minute on med-low heat.)
2. Combine the softened peanut butter and coconut oil with the remaining ingredients in a blender or food processor. Blend until thoroughly combined.
3. Pour into a 9x4" loaf pan that has been lined with parchment paper.
4. Refrigerate until set (about 2 hours).
5. Enjoy.

(Calories 292 | Total Fats 28.9g | Net Carbs: 4.1g | Protein 6g)

Lemon Squares & Coconut Cream

(Total Time: 1 HR 5 MIN| Serve: 8)

Ingredients:

Base:
3/4 cup coconut flakes
2 Tbsp coconut oil
1 Tbsp ground almonds

Cream:
5 eggs
1/2 lemon juice
1 Tbsp coconut flour
1/2 cup stevia sweetener

Directions:

For the base

1. Preheat oven to 360 F.
2. In a bowl, put all base ingredients and mix everything well with clean hands until soft.
3. Grease a rectangle oven dish with coconut oil. Pour dough into a baking pan.
4. Bake for 15 minutes until golden brown. Set aside to cool.

For the cream

5. In a bowl or blender, whisk together eggs, lemon juice, coconut flour, and sweetener. Pour over the baked caked evenly.
6. Put the pan in the oven and bake 20 minutes more.
7. When ready, refrigerate for at least 6 hours. Cut into cubes and serve.

(Calories 129 | Total Fats 15g | Net Carbs: 1.4g | Protein 5g)

Rich Almond Butter Cake & Chocolate Sauce

(Total Time: 10 MIN| **Serve:** 12)

Ingredients:

1 cup almond butter or soaked almonds
1/4 cup almond milk, unsweetened
1 cup coconut oil
2 tsp liquid stevia sweetener to taste

Topping: Chocolate Sauce
4 Tbsp cocoa powder, unsweetened
2 Tbsp almond butter
2 Tbsp stevia sweetener

Directions:

1. Melt the coconut oil in room temperature.
2. Add all ingredients in a bowl and blend well, until combined.
3. Pour the almond butter mixture into a parchment-lined platter.
4. Place in refrigerator for 3 hours.
5. In a bowl, whisk all topping ingredients together. Pour over the almond cake after it's been set. Cut into cubes and serve.

(Calories 273 | Total Fats 23.3g | Net Carbs: 2.4g | Protein 5.8g)

Peanut Butter Cake Covered in Chocolate Sauce

(Total Time: 10 MIN| Serve: 12)

Ingredients:

1 cup peanut butter
1/4 cup almond milk, unsweetened
1 cup coconut oil
2 tsp liquid stevia sweetener to taste

Topping: Chocolate Sauce:
2 Tbsp coconut oil, melted
4 Tbsp cocoa powder, unsweetened
2 Tbsp stevia sweetener

Directions:

1. In a microwave bowl, mix coconut oil and peanut butter; melt in a microwave for 1-2 minutes.
2. Add this mixture to your blender; add in the rest of the ingredients and blend well until combined.
3. Pour the peanut mixture into a parchment-lined loaf pan or platter.
4. Refrigerate for about 3 hours, the longer, the better.
5. In a bowl, whisk all topping ingredients together. Pour over the peanut candy after it's been set. Cut into cubes and serve.

(Calories 273 | Total Fats 27g | Net Carbs: 2.4g | Protein 6g)

Chapter 11: Savory Snacks

Greek-Style Fat Bomb Balls

(Total Time: 15 MIN| **Serve:** 5)

Ingredients:

½ cup cream cheese softened

¼ cup butter softened

3 tsp freshly chopped or dry herbs (any combination of basil, thyme, oregano and/or parsley works great)

4 pieces sun-dried tomatoes, drained

4 kalamata olives, pitted and chopped

2 cloves garlic, crushed

Freshly ground black pepper

¼ tsp sea salt

5 Tbsp parmesan cheese, finely grated

Directions:

1. Mash the butter and cream cheese together with a fork and mix until well combined. Mix in the chopped sun-dried tomatoes and chopped kalamata olives.
2. Add the freshly chopped herbs (or dried), crushed garlic and season with pepper and salt.
3. Mix well and place in refrigerator for 20-30 minutes.
4. Remove the cheese mixture from refrigerator and make 5 balls.
5. Place the grated parmesan cheese in a dish.
6. Coat each ball in the grated parmesan cheese and place on a plate.
7. Serve immediately or store in refrigerator in an airtight container.

(Calories 195 | Total Fats 19.1g | Net Carbs: 2.7g | Protein 4.1g)

Bacon & Onion Cookie Bites

(Total Time: 25 MIN| Serve: 12)

Ingredients:

1 ½ cups almond flour
1/3 cup flax meal
1 Tbsp psyllium husk powder
1 Tbsp onion powder
1 large egg
4 slices bacon, cooked until crispy and crumbled
½ tsp sea salt
Freshly ground pepper

Directions:

1. Place all of the dry ingredients into a bowl and mix until well combined.
2. Add the egg and mix well, using your hands.
3. Add the crumbled bacon to the dough. Process well, using your hands.
4. Using your hands, make 12 equal balls and place them on a baking sheet lined with parchment paper.
5. Use a fork to press and flatten the dough.
6. Place in the oven and bake for 10-12 minutes.
7. When done, the cookies should be golden brown. Remove from oven and cool on a wire rack.
8. Store in a container.
9. Serve and enjoy.

(Calories 151 | Total Fats 12.3g | Net Carbs: 6.1g | Protein 7.3g)

Guacamole & Bacon Fat Bombs

(Total Time: 30 MIN| Serve: 6)

Ingredients:

1 large avocado, halved and peeled
¼ cup butter softened
2 cloves garlic, crushed
1 tsp crushed red pepper
½ small white onion, diced
1 Tbsp fresh lime juice
Freshly ground black pepper
¼ tsp sea salt
4 large slices bacon
2 Tbsp bacon grease, reserved from cooking

Directions:

1. Preheat the oven to 375 F.
2. Line a baking tray with parchment paper. Lay the bacon strips out flat on the parchment paper, leaving space so they don't overlap.
3. Place the tray in the oven and cook for about 10-15 minutes, until golden brown and crisp.
4. When done, remove from the oven and set aside to cool.
5. Place the avocado, butter, crushed red pepper, garlic and lime juice into a bowl and season with pepper and salt.
6. Mash, using masher, until well combined.
7. Add the diced onion and mix well.
8. Pour in the 2 Tbsp of reserved bacon grease and mix well.
9. Cover with foil and place in the refrigerator for 20-30 minutes.
10. Chop the bacon into pieces and place in a dish.
11. Remove the guacamole mixture from refrigerator and make 6 balls.
12. Coat each ball in the bacon crumbles and place on a tray.
13. Serve immediately, or store in the refrigerator in an airtight container for up to 5 days.

(Calories 210 | Total Fats 19.6g | Net Carbs: 4.2g | Protein 5.6g)

Bacon and Egg Fat Bombs

(Total Time: 30 MIN| Serve: 6)

Ingredients:

2 large eggs, hard-boiled, peel and quarter

¼ cup butter softened

2 Tbsp mayonnaise

Freshly ground black pepper

½ tsp sea salt

4 large slices bacon

2 Tbsp bacon grease, reserved from cooking

Directions:

1. Preheat the oven to 375 F.
2. Line a baking tray with parchment paper.
3. Lay the bacon strips out flat on the baking paper, leaving space so they don't overlap.
4. Place the tray in the oven and cook for about 10-15 minutes until golden brown.
5. When done, remove from the oven and set aside to cool down.
6. Cut butter into pieces and add the quartered eggs. Mash with a fork.
7. Add the mayonnaise, season with pepper and salt and mix well.
8. Pour in the bacon grease and mix well.
9. Place in the refrigerator for 20-30 minutes.
10. Chop the bacon into pieces and place in a dish.
11. Remove the egg mixture from refrigerator and make 6 balls.
12. Serve immediately or store in refrigerator in an airtight container for up to 5 days.

(Calories 179 | Total Fats 16.3g | Net Carbs: 1.5g | Protein 6.9g)

Simple Parmesan Crisps

(Total Time: 25 MIN| **Serve:** 4)

Ingredients:

1 cup parmesan cheese

4 Tbsp coconut flour

2 tsp rosemary, oregano or any herbs of choice, dried or fresh

Directions:

1. Preheat the oven to 350 F.
2. In a small bowl, mix the coconut flour, herbs and grated parmesan cheese.
3. Scoop a tsp of the cheese mixture onto a baking tray lined with parchment paper, leaving a small gap between each.
4. Place in preheated oven and cook for 10-15 minutes or until golden brown.
5. Remove from the oven and let the crisps cool down before you remove them from the baking tray.
6. Serve and enjoy.

(Calories 144 | Total Fats 7.5g | Net Carbs: 8.9g | Protein 9.6g)

Mini Pizza Bombs

(Total Time: 10 MIN| **Serve:** 6)

Ingredients:

14 slices Italian sausages

8 pitted black olives

3/4 cup cream cheese

2 Tbsp fresh basil, chopped

2 Tbsp pesto

Salt and pepper to taste

Directions:

1. Dice pitted olives and pepperoni into small pieces.
2. Mix together cream cheese, basil, and pesto.
3. Add the olives and sausage slices into the cream cheese and mix again.
4. Form into balls and garnish with pepperoni, basil, and olive. Ready!!

(Calories 261 | Total Fats 23.43g | Net Carbs: 1g | Protein 10.4g)

Cheesy Bacon Fat Bombs

(Total Time: 15 MIN| **Serve:** 24)

Ingredients:

8 strips cooked crispy bacon, crumbled

1 cup cream cheese, softened

1/2 cup butter

4 tsp bacon fat

4 Tbsp coconut oil

1/4 cup Splenda to taste

Directions:

1. In a microwave dish, combine all ingredients and melt slowly in the microwave until smooth. Set aside some crumbled bacon,
2. Pour into a dish or pan and place in the freezer until firm, about 30 minutes.
3. Before serving, remove from freezer, sprinkle with more crumbled bacon, slice and serve.

(Calories 151 | Total Fats 15.9g | Net Carbs: 0.3g | Protein 0g)

Smoked Turkey, Blue Cheese Eggs

(Total Time: 20 MIN| Serve: 6)

Ingredients:

6 eggs
2 green onions
6 oz smoked turkey breast, chopped
1/2 cup blue cheese, crumbled
2 Tbsp blue cheese dressing
1/4 cup mayonnaise
2 Tbsp hot mustard
1/2 rib celery

Directions:

1. Hard boil the eggs, covered for 12 minutes.
2. In a meanwhile, chop up the smoked turkey breast and the celery.
3. Slice eggs in half lengthwise, scrape the yolks out into a bowl. Add the rest of the ingredients.
4. Grate the green onions over the mixture. Mix all ingredients together.
5. With the tsp, fill every egg with the mixture.
6. Place on a serving plate and refrigerate for one hour. Ready! Serve and enjoy!

(Calories 167 | Total Fats 11.5g | Net Carbs: 0.6g | Protein 14g)

Double Cheese Artichoke Dip

(Total Time: 60 MIN| Serve: 12)

Ingredients:

2 cups artichoke hearts, chopped

16 oz shredded mozzarella cheese

1 cup grated parmesan cheese

1 cup heavy (whipping) cream

1 cup green onion, grated

Directions:

1. Mix all ingredients together and put in a Slow Cooker.
2. Cook on High mode for about one hour.
3. Sprinkle with chopped green onion, if desired.

(Calories 227.64 | Total Fats 15g | Net Carbs: 2.32g | Protein 13.67g)

Easy Artichokes

(Total Time: 2 HR 10 MIN| Serve: 4)

Ingredients:

4 artichokes

3 Tbsp lemon juice

2 Tbsp coconut butter, melted

1 tsp salt and ground black pepper to taste

Water

Directions:

1. Wash and trim artichokes.
2. Start by pulling off the outermost leaves, until you get down to the lighter yellow leaves.
3. Then, using a serrated knife, cut off the top third or so of the artichoke.
4. With the same serrated knife, trim the very bottom of the stem.
5. Mix together salt, melted coconut butter, and lemon juice and pour over artichokes.
6. Pour in water to cover artichokes. Cover and cook on LOW 8hours, or on HIGH 2hours.
7. Serve and enjoy.

(Calories 113.58 | Total Fats 6.98g | Net Carbs: 1.56g | Protein 4.29g)

Pancetta & Eggs

(Total Time: 25 MIN| **Serve:** 4)

Ingredients:

4 large slices pancetta
2 eggs, free-range
1 cup ghee, softened
2 Tbsp mayonnaise
Salt and freshly ground black pepper to taste
Coconut oil for frying

Directions:

1. In a greased non-stick frying pan, bake pancetta on both sides 1-2 minutes. Remove from the heat and set aside.
2. In a meanwhile, boil the eggs. To get the eggs hard-boiled, you need around 10 minutes. When done, wash the eggs well with cold water and peel off the shells.
3. In a deep bowl, place ghee and add the quartered eggs. Mash with a fork. Season it with salt and pepper to taste; add mayonnaise and mix. If you want, you can pour in the pancetta grease. Combine well. Place the bowl in the fridge for one hour at least.
4. Remove the egg mixture from the fridge and make 4 equal balls.
5. Crumble the pancetta into small pieces. Roll each ball in the pancetta crumbles and place on a big platter.
6. Place the egg and pancetta bombs in a fridge for 30 minutes more. Serve cold.

(Calories 238 | Total Fats 22g | Net Carbs: 0.5g | Protein 7.5g)

Parmesan, Herb & Sun-dried Tomato Bombs

(Total Time: 1 HR 20 MIN| Serve: 4)

Ingredients:

1 cup cream cheese
1 cup ghee
5 Tbsp parmesan cheese
1/4 cup sun-dried tomatoes, chopped
1/4 cup kalamata olives, pitted
3 cloves garlic, crushed
3 Tbsp herb mix (basil, parsley, thyme, oregano, parsnip, mint)
Salt and freshly ground black pepper to taste

Directions:

1. In a bowl, combine the cream cheese and ghee. Set aside for 30-45 minutes to soften.
2. Afterwards, mix the ghee and the cream cheese until well combined. Add the chopped kalamata olives and sun-dried tomatoes.
3. Add in herbs and crushed garlic; season with salt and pepper to taste. Mix well with the fork and place bowl in the fridge for at least 1 hour.
4. Remove the cheese mixture from the fridge and create 4 balls. Roll each ball in the grated parmesan cheese and place on a plate.
5. Return it to the fridge for 30 minutes. Serve and enjoy.

(Calories 157 | Total Fats 14g | Net Carbs: 1g | Protein 4.6g)

Cauliflower Tater Tots

(Total Time: 20 MIN| **S**erve: 4)

Ingredients:

1 cauliflower head, cut into florets
2 oz. mozzarella cheese, shredded
¼ cup parmesan cheese, shredded
1 organic egg
½ tsp garlic powder
½ tsp onion powder
2 tsp psyllium husk powder
Salt and pepper to taste
1 cup ghee or lard for frying

Directions:

1. Steam the cauliflower florets.
2. When done, place them in a food processor and process until you achieve a mash. Set aside.
3. Add the mozzarella, parmesan, egg, and the spices into the mixture. Also, add the psyllium husk and then pulse to combine.
4. Using your hands, roll the mixture into small tater tots sizes.
5. Heat the ghee and then fry until golden brown.
6. Allow cooling for a bit, before serving with salsa or sour cream as a dip.

(Calories 249 | Total Fats 21g | Net Carbs: 4g | Protein 10.3 g)

Keto Margherita Pizza

(Total Time: 20 MIN| **Serve:** 2)

Ingredients:

For the crust:
2 organic eggs
2 Tbsp parmesan cheese, grated
1 Tbsp psyllium husk powder
1 tsp Italian seasoning
½ tsp salt
2 tsp ghee

For the toppings:
5 basil leaves, roughly chopped
2 oz. mozzarella cheese, sliced
3 Tbsp all-natural tomato sauce

Directions:

1. Place all the ingredients for the crust in a food processor and pulse until well combined.
2. Pour the mixture into a hot non-stick pan and tilt to spread the batter.
3. Cook until the edges are brown. Flip to the other side and cook for another 45 seconds. Remove from the heat.
4. Spread the tomato sauce on top of the crust, add the mozzarella and basil leaves on top and place in the broiler to melt the cheese for 2 minutes.
5. Serve.

(Calories 459 | Total Fats 35g | Net Carbs: 3.5g | Protein 27g)

Easy Peasy Cheese Pizza

(Total Time: 35 MIN| Serve: 3)

Ingredients:

2 whole eggs
1 cup cheddar cheese, grated
1 Tbsp psyllium husk
3 Tbsp pesto sauce

Directions:

1. Preheat oven to 350 F.
2. Mix eggs and cheese along with the psyllium husk in a bowl and combine well.
3. Place the mixture on baking paper and spread quite thinly. Place in the oven to cook for 15-20 minutes. Remember to keep an eye on it, as it gets brown and crispy quickly relative to the thickness, (don't make it too thin).
4. Once cooked, remove from the oven and place whatever you wish over the base, like the pesto sauce or tomato sauce.
5. Top with your favorite pizza toppings such as bacon slices, pepperoni chicken, fresh tomato, and fresh basil.

(Calories 335 | Total Fats 27g | Net Carbs: 3.2g | Protein 18g)

Keto Trio Queso Quesadilla

(Total Time: 20 MIN| **Serve:** 1)

Ingredients:

¼ cup pepper jack cheese, shredded
¼ cup sharp cheddar cheese, shredded
1 cup mozzarella cheese, cheese
2 Tbsp coconut flour
1 organic egg
½ tsp garlic powder
1 Tbsp almond milk, unsweetened

Directions:

1. Set the oven at 350 F.
2. Microwave the mozzarella in the microwave until it starts to melt.
3. Allow the mozzarella to cool before adding the coconut flour, egg, garlic powder, and milk.
4. Stir well until you achieve a dough-like consistency.
5. Place the dough in between two parchment papers and roll flat.
6. Remove the top parchment paper, transfer the dough to a baking sheet, and place in the oven to bake for 10 minutes.
7. Take out from the oven and allow to cool for a few minutes before topping with the cheeses on one-half of the prepared tortilla.
8. Fold in half and place back in the oven to cook for 5 minutes or until the cheese has melted.

(Calories 977 | Total Fats 73g | Net Carbs: 12g | Protein 63g)

Bacon and Cheese Melt

(Total Time: 15 MIN| **Serve**: 2)

Ingredients:
8 pcs string mozzarella cheese sticks
8 strips of bacon
Olive oil for frying

Directions:
1. Preheat your deep fryer to 350 F.
2. Wrap a cheese stick with one strip of bacon and secure with a toothpick. Repeat until you've used all the bacon and cheese.
3. Deep fry the cheese sticks in the fryer for 3 minutes.
4. Remove and place on top of a paper towel. Serve with a leafy green salad on the side.

(Calories 590 | Total Fats 50g | Net Carbs: 0g | Protein 34g)

BLT Roll

(Total Time: 10 MIN| **Serve**: 1)

Ingredients:
4 leaves, romaine lettuce
4 bacon strips, cooked and crumbled
4 slices deli turkey
1 cup cherry tomatoes cut in half
2 Tbsp mayonnaise

Directions:
1. Lay the turkey slices on top of the lettuce leaves.
2. Spread mayonnaise on the turkey slices and then top with the cherry tomatoes and bacon on top.
3. Roll the lettuce and then secure with a toothpick.
4. Serve immediately.

(Calories 382 | Total Fats 38.5g | Net Carbs: 11.5g | Protein 4.1g)

Portobello Pizza

(Total Time: 25 MIN| **Serve:** 4)

Ingredients:

1 medium tomato, sliced
¼ cup basil, chopped
20 pepperoni slices
4 Portobello mushroom caps
4 oz mozzarella cheese
6 Tbsp olive oil
Black pepper
Salt

Directions:

1. Remove insides of mushrooms and take out meat, so that the shell is left.
2. Coat mushrooms with half of oil and season with pepper and salt; broil for 5 minutes then turn over and coat with leftover oil. Bake for an additional 5 minutes.
3. Add tomato to the inside of shell and top with basil, pepperoni, and cheese. Broil for 4 minutes until cheese melts.
4. Serve warm.

(Calories 321 | Total Fats 31g | Net Carbs: 2.8g | Protein 8.5g)

Basil and Bell Pepper Pizza

(Total Time: 30 MIN| Serve: 2)

Ingredients:

For Base:
½ cup almond flour
2 tsp cream cheese
1 egg
½ tsp salt
6 oz mozzarella cheese
2 Tbsp psyllium husk
2 Tbsp parmesan cheese
1 tsp Italian seasoning
½ tsp black pepper

For Toppings:
1 medium tomato, sliced
2/3 bell pepper, sliced
4 oz cheddar cheese, shredded
¼ cup tomato sauce
3 Tbsp basil, chopped

Directions:

1. Preheat oven to 400 F. Place mozzarella into a microwave safe dish and melt for 1 minute, stirring occasionally.
2. Add cream cheese to melted mozzarella and combine.
3. Mix dry ingredients for base together in a bowl, add egg and combine. Add cheese mixture and use hands to combine into a dough.
4. Form dough into a circle, bake for 10 minutes and remove from oven. Top with tomato sauce, tomato, basil, bell pepper and cheddar cheese.
5. Return to oven and bake for 10 additional minutes.
6. Serve warm.

(Calories 410 | Total Fats 31.3g | Net Carbs: 5.3g | Protein 24.8g)

Chapter 12: Smoothies

Blueberry Almond Smoothie

(Total Time: 12 MIN| Serve: 2)

Ingredients:

16 oz almond milk, unsweetened

1 tsp xylitol

4 oz heavy cream

¼ cup frozen unsweetened blueberries

1 scoop whey vanilla protein powder

Directions:

1. Put all ingredients in a blender and blend until smooth.
2. Add a little water if it becomes too thick.
3. Measure those blueberries as they add more carbs.

(Calories 314 | Total Fats 23.7g | Net Carbs: 8.7g | Protein 16.4g)

Choco-Cashew Orange Smoothie

(Total Time: 10 MIN| Serve: 1)

Ingredients:

1 cup cashew milk

1 handful of arugula leaves

1 Tbsp chocolate whey protein powder

1/8 tsp orange extract

Ice cubes

Directions:

1. Place all ingredients in your blender and blend until well united and smooth.
2. Add extra ice and serve.

(Calories 45 | Total Fats 1.05g | Net Carbs: 7g | Protein 3g)

Strawberry Majoram Smoothie

(Total Time: 10 MIN| Serve: 1)

Ingredients:

1/4 cup fresh or frozen strawberries

2 fresh marjoram leaves

2 Tbsp heavy cream

1 cup unsweetened coconut milk

1 Tbsp sugar-free vanilla syrup

1/2 tsp pure vanilla extract

Ice cubes

Directions:
1. Place all ingredients in your blender and mix until become smooth.
2. If you wish you can add the ice cubes. Serve for a refreshing summer drink.

(Calories 292 | Total Fats 26.7g | Net Carbs: 6g | Protein 2.8g)

The Green Fuel

(Total Time: 10 MIN| Serve: 1)

Ingredients:

1 cup almond milk, unsweetened

1 cup baby spinach

½ ripe avocados

½ Tbsp stevia

1 cup ice

Directions:
1. Place all the ingredients into a blender and blend until smooth.
2. Serve and consume immediately.

(Calories 382 | Total Fats 38.5g | Net Carbs: 11.5g | Protein 4.1g)

Beet Cucumber Smoothie

(Total Time: 10 MIN| Serve: 4)

Ingredients:

1 cup spinach leaves

2 cups cucumber (peeled, seeded and chopped)

1/2 cup carrot chopped

1/2 cup fresh beetroot

3/4 cup heavy (whipping) cream

4 tsp sweetener of your choice (optional)

Handful of ground almonds

1 cup ice cubes

1 cup water

Directions:

1. Place all ingredients in a blender.
2. Pulse until smooth. Serve immediately.

(Calories 137.91 | Total Fats 12.99g | Net Carbs: 3.4g | Protein 1.66g)

Green Devil Smoothie

(Total Time: 10 MIN| Serve: 2)

Ingredients:

3 cup kale, fresh

1/2 cup coconut yogurt

1/2 cup broccoli, florets

2 celery stalk, chopped

2 cup water

1 Tbsp lemon juice

Ice cubes (if needed)

Directions:

1. Blend all ingredients together until smooth and slightly frothy.
2. Enjoy!

(Calories 117.09 | Total Fats 4.98g | Net Carbs: 1.89g | Protein 4.09g)

Cilantro and Ginger Smoothie

(Total Time: 10 MIN| Serve: 3)

Ingredients:

1/2 cup fresh cilantro (chopped)

2-inch ginger, fresh

1 cucumber

2 Tbsp chia seeds

1/2 cup spinach, fresh

1 Tbsp almond butter

Handful of ground almonds

1 lime (or lemon)

2 cups water

Directions:

1. Blend spinach, cucumber, and water until smooth.
2. Add the remaining fruits and blend again, before serving.

(Calories 102.72 | Total Fats 6.92g | Net Carbs: 13.96g | Protein 71g)

Green Coconut Smoothie

(Total Time: 10 MIN| Serve: 2)

Ingredients:

1 cup coconut milk

1 green apple, cored and chopped

1 cup spinach

1 cucumber

2 Tbsp shaved coconut

1/2 cup water

Ice cubes (if needed)

Directions:

1. Put all ingredients and ice in a blender; pulse until smooth.
2. Serve immediately.

(Calories 216.57 | Total Fats 16.56g | Net Carbs: 8.79g | Protein 2.88g)

Green Dream Keto Smoothie

(Total Time: 10 MIN| Serve: 4)

Ingredients:

1 cup raw cucumber, peeled and sliced

4 cups water

1 cup romaine lettuce

1 cup Haas avocado

2 Tbsp fresh basil

Sweetener of your choice (optional)

Handful of walnuts

2 Tbsp fresh parsley

1 Tbsp fresh ginger grated

Ice cubes (optional)

Directions:

1. In a blender, combine all of the ingredients and pulse until smooth. Add ice. Serve cold.

(Calories 50.62| Total Fats 3.89g | Net Carbs: 1.07g | Protein 1.1g)

Almond Choc Shake

(Total Time: 5 MIN| Serve: 2)

Ingredients:

16 oz almond milk, unsweetened

1 tbsp chia seeds

1 tsp xylitol

½ tsp cacao powder

4 oz heavy cream

1 scoop whey chocolate isolate powder

1/2 cup crushed ice

Directions:

1. Add all ingredients into the blender and blend until smooth.

(Calories 292 | Total Fats 25g | Net Carbs: 4g | Protein 15.27g)

Keto Celery and Nut Smoothie

(Total Time: 10 MIN| Serve: 2)

Ingredients:

2 celery stem
1 cup spinach leaves, roughly chopped
1/2 cup pistachio nuts (unsalted)
1/2 avocado, chopped
1/2 cup lime, juice
1 Tbsp hemp seeds
1 Tbsp almonds, soaked
1 cup coconut water
Ice cubes (optional)

Directions:

1. Add all ingredients in a blender with a few ice cubes and blend until smooth.

(Calories 349.55 | Total Fats 17.88g | Net Carbs: 5.01g | Protein 11.08g)

Coco and Blueberry Smoothie

(Total Time: 5 MIN| Serve: 2)

Ingredients:

½ cup blueberries
½ cup coconut cream
1 Tbsp coconut oil
½ cup almond milk, vanilla flavor
3 ice cubes

Directions:

1. Place all the ingredients in a blender and mix until you achieve a smooth consistency.

(Calories 237 | Total Fats 21.9g | Net Carbs: 12.1g | Protein 1.9g)

Lime Peppermint Smoothie

(Total Time: 5 MIN| Serve: 4)

Ingredients:
1/4 cup fresh mint leaves
1/4 cup lime juice
1/2 cup cucumber, chopped
1 Tbsp fresh basil leaves, chopped
1 tsp chia seed (optional)
Handful of chia seeds
3 tsp zest of limes
Sweetener of your choice to taste
1 cup water, divided
Ice as needed

Directions:
1. Place all ingredients in a blender or food processor. Pulse until smooth well.
2. Fill glasses with ice, pour the limeade into each glass, and enjoy.

(Calories 28.11 | Total Fats 1.16g | Net Carbs: 0.75g | Protein 0.84g)

Berry Breakfast Shake

(Total Time: 5 MIN| Serve: 1)

Ingredients:
¾ cup mixed berries
1 cup almond milk
1 Tbsp all-natural peanut butter
1 Tbsp protein powder
¼ tsp cinnamon powder
¼ tsp ginger, minced

Directions:
1. Add all the ingredients in a blender and blend until smooth.

(Calories 319 | Total Fats 15g | Net Carbs: 9g | Protein 28g)

Red Grapefruit Kale Smoothies

(Total Time: 10 MIN| Serve: 4)

Ingredients:

2 cups cantaloupe

1/4 cup fresh strawberries

8 oz coconut yogurt

2 cups kale leaves, chopped

2 Tbsp sweetener of your taste

1 Ice as needed

1 cup water

Directions:

1. Clean the grapefruit and remove the seeds.
2. Combine all ingredients in an electric blender and whirl until smooth. Add ice and serve.

(Calories 260.74 | Total Fats 11.57g | Net Carbs: 2.96g | Protein 4.42g)

Simple Keto Avocado Smoothie

(Total Time: 10 MIN| Serve: 2)

Ingredients:

2.6 oz avocado

2 cup water

2 tsp chia seeds

0.5 oz fresh spinach

2 fl oz heavy whipping cream

1 tsp vanilla extract, unsweetened

1 Tbsp extra virgin coconut oil

Liquid stevia extract

Few ice cubes

Directions:

1. First, bisect the avocado. Carefully remove thepip.
2. In a blender, put all ingredients, sweetener and the ice (if used) and beat until smooth. Serve.

(Calories 226.44 | Total Fats 23.63g | Net Carbs: 0.18g | Protein 1.66g)

Vanilla Protein Smoothie

(Total Time: 5 MIN| Serve: 2)

Ingredients:

1 cup baby spinach

5 Tbsp of heavy cream

3 Tbsp organic nut butter of your choice

1/2 cup vanilla protein powder

3 Tbsp sweetener of your choice

1 cup of water

Ice cubes

Directions:

1. Place all ingredients in a blender and pulse until smooth well.
2. Serve with ice cubes (optional).

(Calories 256.18 | Total Fats 21.79g | Net Carbs: 3.88g | Protein 8.41g)

Keto Avocado Smoothie

(Total Time: 7 MIN| Serve: 3)

Ingredients:

1 Haas avocado

3 oz almond milk, unsweetened

3 oz heavy whipping cream

6 drops liquid stevia

Ice cubes

Directions:

1. Cut the avocado in half, remove the pip and remove the flesh from the skin.
2. In a blender, mix the almond milk, avocado, heavy whipping cream, sweetener and ice cubes. Blend 1 minute and serve.

(Calories 252.92 | Total Fats 24.43g | Net Carbs: 8.31g | Protein 3.69g)

Caramel Coffee Smoothie

(Total Time: 5 MIN| Serve: 4)

Ingredients:

1/2 cup heavy cream

1/2 cup almond milk, unsweetened

3 Tbsp sugar-free chocolate syrup

3 Tbsp sugar-free caramel syrup

3/4 cup cold coffee

2 Tbsp cocoa, unsweetened

Ice cubes

Directions:

1. In a blender add all ingredients and blend until all incorporated well.
2. Pour into glasses and serve.

(Calories 170.62 | Total Fats 14.95g | Net Carbs: 9.02g | Protein 2.8g)

Creamy Chocolate Milk

(Total Time: 12 MIN| Serve: 2)

Ingredients:

16 oz almond milk, unsweetened

1 tsp xylitol

4 oz heavy cream

1 scoop whey chocolate isolates powder

½ cup crushed ice (optional)

Directions:

1. Put all ingredients in a blender and blend until smooth.
2. This recipe can be doubled, as can most low carb smoothie recipes.

(Calories 292 | Total Fats 25g | Net Carbs: 4g | Protein 15g)

Conclusion
Thank for downloading this book!

I hope that you will use what you've learned from this book on your journey to lose weight, and most importantly, become healthier. Yes, there are many diets out there that promise the same results, however, the Ketogenic Diet is one of the few that is scientifically proven and truly works!

Remember, losing weight doesn't mean that you have to skip your meals and starve yourself in order to lose weight. What you just need to do is to watch what you eat—limit your carbs, moderately consume protein, and eat more fat - the healthy type of fat!

The Ketogenic Diet will help you achieve your health goals, but just like any other diets, your commitment and perseverance to follow this diet is needed for you to reap its benefits. Use the tips, recipes, and meal plans that I shared with you during the first weeks of your Keto Diet. Also, don't be afraid to explore other recipes that you wish to include in your meal plan. As long as you stay within the numbers of the required macros you need to consume, then you're assured that your body will continuously burn fat.

Try the Ketogenic diet and gain mental clarity, burn excess fat and have unlimited energy today. I wish you great health and good tidings as you set out on this amazing journey to ultimate health.

All the best!

Finally, if you feel that you have received any value from this book, then I'd like to ask if you would be kind enough to click on the link below and leave a review on Amazon to share your positive experience with other readers.
It'd be greatly appreciated!

69883001R00248

Made in the USA
Lexington, KY
06 November 2017